GETTING DOCTORED

GETTING DOCTORED

Critical reflections on becoming a physician

MARTIN SHAPIRO, M.D.

between the lines

© 1978 Martin Shapiro

Published by: Between the Lines
97 Victoria Street North,
Kitchener, Ontario, Canada

Typeset by: Dumont Press Graphix
Kitchener, Ontario, Canada

Cover drawing by: Michal Manson

Printed and bound in Canada by:
The Hunter Rose Company

Between the Lines receives financial assistance from the Ontario Arts Council.

Canadian Cataloguing in Publication Data

Shapiro, Martin.
  Getting doctored

ISBN 0-919946-10-0 bd. ISBN 0-919946-09-7 pa.

1. Medical students. 2. Medical education.
I. Title.

R737.S53   610'.739   C79-094103-1

This book is dedicated to those Chilean health workers who struggled to transform their society and died at the hands of the government which took power in the coup of September 11, 1973.

Acknowledgements

In the writing of this book I received considerable moral, intellectual and emotional support from a number of individuals. I can mention only a few of them here, but there were many more whose help was invaluable.

Sam Abramovitch furnished much-needed encouragement to me in the idea of writing a book, and criticized the work section by section as I wrote. Donald Bates, Veda Charrow, Sheldon Greenfield, Russell Jacoby, Joseph Lella and Jeremy Walker recommended readings in their respective areas of expertise and provided helpful and constructive critiques of the preliminary drafts. Approximately twenty other persons read and criticized the book in ways that enabled me to improve it significantly. Lynn Bevan and Josh Freed were instrumental in my connecting with Between the Lines as a publisher and thus introducing me to the comradely solidarity that I received from the people who work there. Their commitment to progressive social action through productive activity will always be a model for me. I was most fortunate to have Nick Sullivan and Robert Clarke as editors. They shared my vision of what this book should be and unflinchingly devoted considerable time and their remarkable talents to making it clearer and more accessible. I can only admire the patience they demonstrated towards the idiosyncrasies of a writer while we worked together. Notwithstanding all this very important aid which I received, it is I who must bear responsibility for whatever errors, inconsistencies and inadequacies remain in the book.

When it has seemed appropriate, I have quoted from other works. These quotations are easily recognizable by smaller type or enclosure in quotation marks. They are cited in all cases as references, and all are from copyrighted works; they may not be reproduced elsewhere without permission from the respective publishers.

This book was supported in part by a grant from the Robert Wood Johnson Foundation and by stipends from the Department of Medicine, Royal Victoria Hospital, Montreal. It should be obvious from what follows that the views expressed and conclusions reached are my own and in no way reflect the views of these organizations or their officials.

Martin Shapiro
Los Angeles
December, 1978

Contents

References:

Reference notes to articles and books are indicated by superior numbers (e.g. [24]) throughout the text. These notes are listed at the end of the book under the chapter in which the reference appears.

Asterisks (*) refer to explanatory notes. They are listed at the back of each chapter according to the page number on which they appear.

Preface

When I entered medical school at McGill University, Montreal, in 1969, student activism and the influence of the "new left" were at their peak. McGill itself had witnessed the student occupation of two campus buildings in the previous two years. Many Great Issues were being debated energetically: the student's role in the university, the war in Vietnam, the role of the university in effecting social change, the organization of society. Every medical student was aware of these debates and a number of my classmates—perhaps a dozen—were openly sympathetic to people within the university who were challenging established values.

Long before I had finished the medical course, most of this awareness, sympathy and activism had vanished. This was, of course, part of a trend in the seventies: students were spending less time thinking about problems outside their own lives. But the members of my medical class seemed to be undergoing a much more thorough transformation than could be written off as a trend of the times. The change seemed closely related to the process we had undergone in our studies, the systems we had learned, the specializations and the expectations we had driven into us, all usually quite willingly. In other words, it was part of the process of socialization inherent in becoming a doctor.

Compounding my concern for this transition of apparently nice people into Doctors (who are frequently not nice at all) was a growing awareness of many disturbing aspects of social interactions in hospitals as well as in medical school.

By the end of my final year, I had already given considerable thought to the possibility of putting something down on paper about what my colleagues and I were experiencing. During the year after graduation, while I was interning and preparing to receive my licence to practise, the project became much clearer in my mind: the next year would be devoted to writing a book on the process of being socialized into the role of physician.

I was aware of the many available books on various aspects of medical education, training and practice; I had read a number of them. To the extent that I sought in them answers to questions troubling me, I found none satisfactory. The most simplistic and objectionable of them attempted to whitewash medicine, portraying a process far less brutal and far more humane than the reality I knew (although even in these books the real world still managed to sneak in and rear its ugly head occasionally). Most of these medical fairy tales were written by physicians.

Other books acknowledged the existence of serious problems, but each of them ascribed all the ills of medical practice and medical education to One Underlying Problem: physicians are too greedy; the hours of interning are too long; the medical profession conceals its blunders; medical school destroys the idealism of the future physician; or whatever. In each case, The Problem was postulated as the rate-limiting step in a process where the basic chemistry remained unchallenged. Physicians wrote some of these tracts too, although many came from the pens of social scientists. Nothing I read looked systematically at medicine in society. The books lacked a recognition that many of the problems of medicine are palpably linked to problems in society as a whole.*

Then along came Ivan Illich, who did propose such a connection. In his widely read book *Medical Nemisis*,[1] Illich resoundingly affirms the importance of the relationship between medicine and society, which he conceives to operate approximately thus: medical institutions and medical practitioners oppress people; dependence on medical care deprives people of the capacity for autonomous activity in all aspects of their lives, and not merely when they are ill. This notion, that medicine is responsible for social problems, is called *structural iatrogenesis* by Illich. It is, in reality, the *reductio ad absurdum* of the thesis — implicitly shared by the authors referred to above — that society is not to blame for medicine's ills. Illich goes so far as to assert that people can begin to emancipate themselves from the many oppressive influences in their lives by throwing off the medical yoke.

A review of the literature convinced me that my undertaking was worthwhile, both for self-clarification and as a contribution to the remarkably underdeveloped discussion.[2] I began by researching a number of issues that already concerned me. I set out with no readymade answers and a few preconceptions, but I did have some perspective: I believed it unlikely that problems in medicine could be adequately explained if one attempted to abstract them from their social context. I commenced by rereading some previously encountered literature that had seemed relevant in various ways to my medical experience. I also sought the guidance of others in selecting appropriate reading materials.

As I worked my way through my inventory of problems (and became better able to self-direct my reading), it became apparent that *none* of the issues that concerned me could be studied adequately in isolation from the rest. I came to recognize that problems such as the competitiveness in medical school, the hierarchy of the hospital, and the physician-patient relationship, are in fact closely related to each other and to society as a whole. I found some concepts especially useful in illuminating these relationships. In particular, Karl Marx's theory of alienation helped me to make sense of many difficult areas. I had already read some of Marx's writings; it was not until I sat down to reflect critically on my life in medicine, however, that I began to recognize the rich contributions of his system to the comprehension of human experience. I saw much in medicine that seemed to manifest the alienation Marx described.

I also found that Erich Fromm's writings on the subject of authoritarianism made some problems more intelligible. Fromm suggests that in certain groups within society, authoritarian interaction can be particularly prevalent. It struck me that authoritarianism is in fact very much the norm in medical settings from the first day of medical school, through hospital experience, right into office practice.

The book that results from this work is an exploration of a series of medical problems related to medical education (both in medical schools and in hospitals) and to the practice of medicine in North American university-affiliated hospitals. In many ways it is a personal exploration: I have endeavoured to illustrate these problems with events drawn from my own experience, and these events are points of reference for my analysis. I do this in order that readers can encounter the concepts used in the book as I did, at times and in ways that affirm their validity and relevance. In this sense, the book might be called a "critical memoir". I have also tried to provide a partial resume of current debate, when it exists, on each topic as it arises. At the same time I emphasize that the problems raised are both related to one another and to problems and factors outside of the medical context. *Getting Doctored* thus moves from the question of how students get into medical school in the first place, to the different kinds of teaching and socialization processes they confront while there, to what happens when they reach the hospital wards. The book looks also at the hierarchy of relationships established in hospitals and the kind of patient-doctor relationships that result. There are also chapters dealing with the special effect of increasing technology and specialization on medical practice and the effect of medical jargon on the social level.

As the writing proceeded, it became apparent to me that the questions of alienation and authoritarianism in medicine demanded separate consideration. Consequently, I have ended the book with a chapter devoted exclusively to these concepts, without particular reference to my own experience but drawing together many of the points of exploration earlier in the book.

When I had written the first draft of the book, I returned to medical work as a resident in internal medicine (the final phase of my medical training and which I have just now completed). I was then able to test my model against what I actually encountered in the hospital. My experiences as a resident in both Montreal and Los Angeles — and the problems were strikingly similar in the two cities — taught me much that was incorporated in subsequent revisions.

In the end, I most deliberately do not propose any panaceas. I have learned, however, that the only productive way to examine social problems, whether they *seem* to be situated in a medical setting or anywhere else, is in relation to the totality of society. Using this approach, one perceives the need to transcend the confines of any particular discipline or framework of analysis. The problems dealt with by sociology, psychology, philosophy, economics, politics and history are but different faces of the one problem of our social existence.

I do not explore these many disciplines equally in this book. Economics, for example, is dealt with in a relatively peripheral way. What I *have* tried to do is to draw on each field to the extent necessary to develop my argument. This method makes apparent, I think, the unity of a process that extends well beyond the material I actually discuss.

In this spirit, I have not directed my writing to a narrow audience in either the occupational or the ideological sense. Instead, I have used as my point of departure Bertolt Brecht's maxim: "We must address not only people who hold certain views, but people who, because of their situation, should hold these views."[3]

My understanding of the issues is continuing to evolve. I have no illusion that the definitive statement on any of the problems raised is to be found here. On the contrary, in the process of writing I have become convinced of the need to undertake further researches on many of them. I do hope to dispel for some the notion that solutions can be found to problems in medicine when these are considered *as* merely 'problems in medicine'.

If this book contributes to the growth of an emphasis on looking at problems in relation to the whole of society, then I shall have accomplished something useful. The public discussions of medicine and society are in need of such a reorientation.

Notes

page 8: I have not yet had an opportunity to evaluate Vincente Navarro's book *Medicine Under Capitalism* (New York: Neil Watson Academic Publisher, 1977), which seems to be an exception.

Criticism is an act of love.

— slogan printed on a wall
in San Francisco, February, 1973

1

Getting In

Where do doctors come from? Or, who goes to medical school and how do they get there?

My high school class in Winnipeg might serve as an example. Geographically, the school straddled middle class and working class districts. My own class, however, comprised thirty students with the highest grades in the school: needless to say, we were all from the "right side of the tracks". Now, as I look back on that class, I realize that the aspirations of the students were remarkably uniform. Coming mainly from middle class families, we never had any doubts that our paths would lead straight through one of the professions. All of us were encouraged by our parents, overtly or otherwise, in this direction. Some made minor modifications in their ambitions, by choice or necessity, but the general outcome of the pursuit of career in that class was never really in doubt. At last count, we had produced three academics, five physicians and six lawyers.

During high school I knew of several students in my class who were intent on becoming physicians to the exclusion of all else (they were all male; I do not recall any women sharing this "dream"). One of them, for instance, talked of little else during his high school years, in spite of not being particularly proficient in science studies. It seemed he could not imagine himself as becoming anything else; his older brother was already a doctor.

"Do you think I'll get into medicine?" he would ask. "I don't know what I'll do if I don't. There's nothing else I want to be."

Three other students in my class who had medical school ambitions were themselves the sons of physicians. One had rather mediocre grades; it turned out he had to apply two or three times before getting in. Another had quite broad interests; he later dropped out of medical school after a week, drifted around a bit and ended up as a lawyer. The third never had any doubts about where he was heading and is now a cardiologist.

Is this middle class scenario in which I partook representative?

In general, medical students in North America are recruited from the economically privileged sectors of society. Over a decade ago, Canada's Royal Commission on Health Services reported that 54.4 per cent of general practitioners and 65.8 per cent of specialists in Canada, at the time of their entry into university, had fathers with professional or managerial occupations. In addition, 73 per cent of all physicians had fathers whose occupational class, according to one index, was among the top 17 per cent in the country; fifteen per cent of Canadian physicians have doctors for parents.[1] The pattern is similar in the United States, where 58 per cent of physicians come from professional or managerial backgrounds and about 17 per cent have physician parents.[2]

Of 135 students in my medical course at McGill University, Montreal, I knew ten (and there were probably more) whose fathers were physicians. There were at least three in the class who were children of the elite (one was the son of the president of a large trust company, another was the son of the president of a large pharmaceutical company and the third was the daughter of the President of Liberia). Only a handful of students were from working class families, and just one from a family that was genuinely poor. The rest were from the various strata of the middle class and upwards. In this sense, we were probably representative of most medical school rosters today. We had a "relatively homogeneous social background",[3] and few of us would have been thought destined for "lesser" careers.

Enthusiastic, hard-working and bright, without a doubt, but the collegians who made it into medical school were of a different and finer slice of society than were those who did not, just as the movement from high school to college left behind many of the children of the working class. What was perhaps most remarkable about us (and about those with whom we competed for admission) was the extent to which it mattered that we get in.

The scramble for admission

Certainly one of the reasons for wanting to follow a medical career is an economic one: as one admissions officer said, "Medicine is almost the only career that offers total security." In fact, medicine is one of the very few professions in our society in which the worker has absolute job security, at least in the last couple of decades. Physicians can always find work, whatever their clients, fellow workers and even bosses (when they exist) think of them. Physicians are also respected in the community in a way that few other people are. There is ample (some would say excessive) economic return for their labours; a doctor's income is sufficient to provide an effective buffer against economic downturns, stagflation and all the rest. The work itself is often gratifying, interesting and stimulating. All these factors combine to make the life of "Doctor" an oasis — or at least the mirage of one — in a desert of unhappy work and life experiences. All students entering medical school are aware of this.

It is not really surprising, then, that students from privileged backgrounds end up in this kind of professional career. The expectations of parents, for one thing, play an important role. My parents never openly urged me to go to medical school, but they did discourage a career in journalism. I suppose it was my acceptance of a set of values stressing economic security that made it probable I would end up in something like medicine.

Once the decision to attend a medical school is made, the process of applying is tortuous. McGill had an officer whose full-time job was to advise students about entering medical schools. If such a person is not around to tell students how to go about applying and to offer a realistic assessment of their prospects, the situation can be even more anxiety-provoking than it is. In order to apply to just one medical school, students have to complete the appropriate application forms, pay a fee, forward their undergraduate grades, write a standardized quiz (the Medical College Admission Test), arrange for letters of recommendation to be sent and, finally, submit to one or more interviews.

Then too, because acceptance at any one medical school is rarely guaranteed, almost all students serious about applying submit applications to several. Not infrequently one encounters the determined character who has applied to each of the more than 100 schools in North America. This multiple application process of course builds up the numbers considered for entrance at different universities and thereby makes the apparent odds longer for any one student at any one particular school. This only increases the applicants' anxiety and provokes even more applications. At McGill, some three thousand students (and the figure is still climbing) apply each year for the one hundred and sixty positions open, so the competition is intense.*

The scramble for admissions at McGill is embodied in a "premedical society", made up of students pragmatically working together, covering all the angles in their bids to become physicians. These students develop contacts which will later be useful as references; they learn of the obstacles in the admissions ordeal; perhaps most important, they structure this critical period in their lives so they can at least draw strength from the experience of others.

It is all a serious business: students who engage in premedical societies and other rituals intended to improve their chances of getting in would probably do so even if the activity made no difference to their chances. Persons who call themselves premedical students, whatever their prospects for subsequent acceptance, are engaged in a kind of dance of destiny. By acting out the role of premedical student, they hope to identify themselves as such. If they bow early and often before the altar of medicine, they may just obtain the salvation that they associate with admission to medical school and a medical career.

How to get in

What factors govern the student's chances of getting in?

"Only two things really matter: marks and pull", one member of McGill's admissions committee told me.

Academic performance is perhaps the most important determinant of a student's chances. And while this particular determinant may not discriminate in favour of the privileged few, it does tend to militate *against* those who, for one reason or another, have not excelled in their undergraduate courses.

Excelling, by present-day medical school standards, means that the individual must obtain top marks consistently throughout the undergraduate years. The competition for places in the medical class is so fierce that an admissions committee doesn't have to settle for anyone who is, by this criterion, second best. That means students who have, for instance, taken time out to question their role in society and place in the university, allowing "performance" to suffer as a result, or who have changed interests (and courses) in midstream, may be at a disadvantage: they may have failed to demonstrate that they are above all "good students" and "know what they want".

Many students, on the other hand, faithfully tailor their undergraduate programme to appeal to members of admissions committees. Some deliberately choose not to take courses in the humanities which otherwise interest them, precisely because they fear not obtaining the obligatory "A" grade.[4] This obsession with grades sometimes leads to strange situations. One professor, not at all atypical, reports that fifty students invariably line up outside his office the day after he posts the grades in his biology course; the students hope to garner the extra point or two that might make the difference between an acceptable and an inadequate average. These students are pursuing not an education, but a position in a medical school class, and their undergraduate professors are, in a very real sense, sitting in judgement as to whether or not their disciples should be allowed to go on to the coveted goal. Understandably, many professors are unhappy with this role.

The other factor in the entrance equation is "pull" and there is no doubt that some people have a great deal more going for them than others. One McGill admissions committee member reports having received a telephone call from the Prime Minister of Canada urging that a particular student be accepted. Another tells of an anxious father who phoned and said, "If you accept my son, I'll deposit $10,000 in your bank account tomorrow." Occasionally such incidents seep into public awareness, creating shock and indignation, as when it was reported that at least eight students gained admission to the medical school at the University of California's Davis campus because of wealth or good connections.[5]

In both of the McGill cases, I was told, the intervention did not influence the committee deliberations. Nevertheless, there are certainly some institutions where pressure, perhaps more subtly applied, has some effect on the candidate's chances. Reflecting on this, one admissions committee member remarked: "It is often difficult to say no to your colleagues."

Cronyism — favouring the sons of fellow physicians, of university professors, and of others the committee member knows — is probably responsible, at least in part, for the fact that fifteen per cent of Canadian physicians and seventeen per cent of American physicians have physician parents. Certainly, in comparison with the proportion of physicians in the population, much larger numbers of physicians' children are getting into medical school than would be likely in an entirely meritocratic system.

How not to get in

Students from backgrounds that do not encourage academic achievement, or from social situations in which university attendance (and, even more, professional ambition) is not the norm, or from backgrounds in which, for various reasons, the preparation for university has been inadequate, will be at a serious disadvantage in the competition for positions in the medical class, even if they do apply.*

The priority given to academic standing is a form of discrimination against the poor. One expression of this is under-representation in medical schools of those minorities who are over-represented in the lower socio-economic groups. There were no black Canadians or black Americans in my class. (There were a few Africans, all from wealthy families.) There were also no native people, in spite of the fact that our school had been very self-congratulatory about its efforts to supply medical personnel to the Canadian north, which receives such inadequate medical service.

Some groups have begun to agitate for greater representation in medical classes. American blacks, who had been virtually shut out of white medical schools (there are two black schools: Howard and Meharry), have been admitted in growing numbers in the last few years.[6] As yet, no such organized efforts have been undertaken to better represent the poor.* Most positions at medical schools remain the preserve of the meritocracy, which is often resentful of even the token concessions made to minorities. ("I can only compete for 115 of 130 positions in the Harvard medical class," a Boston area student told me.) Even the existing program, however, has been straining the American legal and constitutional apparatus. An applicant rejected by a medical school in California has successfully contended before the courts that he was "improperly denied" a place in medical school when positions were given to "less qualified" minority applicants.[7]*

Another practice of medical school admissions committees is to limit severely the number of places open to foreigners. Very few medical schools admit any foreigners at all. McGill is one exception. My class had 32 non-Canadians, almost 25 per cent of the total students. Of these, however, 20 were Americans and, of the remaining 12, virtually all were from families wealthy in their native lands. In 1972, a total of 240 foreign nationals were admitted to American medical schools, an average of less than three per school. There were, on the other hand, 3715 Americans registered at all levels in overseas medical schools the same year.[8] Many of these eventually return to practise in the United States; the training of a physician is an expensive proposition, and this amounts, in effect, to a subsidization of North American medical education by less prosperous countries.[9]

Political discrimination is undoubtedly widespread in the selection of the few foreigners who do get into the medical schools. One member of my class, who was from the Far East, was asked during one of four pre-admission interviews at McGill what he thought of the Domino Theory! An interviewer at the University of Southern California asked the same applicant what side he would fight for in a war between the United States and China.

But the political views of non-foreign students may be a factor in admissions as well. Although politics did not come up in my own interview, some of my classmates reported that they were questioned about their views on universal health insurance (Medicare) and the Saskatchewan doctors' strike; these questions came from committee members who seemed antagonistic to societal interventions in the delivery of medical care. They may have felt they had good reason: the class prior to ours had included a number of leftward-leaning individuals who had given headaches to the faculty by questioning health care priorities and the medical school curriculum. This behaviour on the part of the usually docile students upset many faculty members; they considered it a mistake to have allowed such people into medical school. The head of the admissions committee was relieved of his responsibilities, reportedly because of this "error". Needless to say, the admissions committee was more careful in its selections for my year, resulting in a much more conservative class. At a time when campus radicalism was at its peak, the number of "progressive" minds in my class was relatively small.*

One innovation in admissions policy the year I applied was a marked increase in the number of French Canadians accepted. In the three previous years a total of seven had been admitted; in my year there were eighteen. Some of the Francophone members of the class reported that they had three or four separate interviews during the admissions process. No Anglophone student I have spoken to had this experience.

There had been some agitation around that time to convert the university to French language use. "We were careful to choose French boys who were quite conservative," a committee member told me. "We didn't want any trouble."

Women and admissions

Yet another form of discrimination restricts the number of women who are permitted to embark on medical training, and the struggle of women to obtain a significant proportion of positions in medical classes in North American schools has been arduous. Only Spain has a smaller proportion of female to male physicians than have Canada and the United States.[10] In recent years there has been an upswing in female enrolment but this has not yet made much of a dent in the physician work force.[11]

Of course at one time things were much worse. McGill did not graduate any women physicians at all until 1922.[12] Harvard's medical school, even worse, did not graduate a woman until 1949.[13] The Johns Hopkins Medical School in Baltimore was an exception: it admitted women from its founding in 1889, apparently motivated by a substantial donation from four Baltimore women "under the expressed condition that women be admitted . . . on an equal footing with men".[14]

An early incident at McGill is indicative of the pressures against female enrolment.[15] In 1888, a woman named Grace Ritchie was the valedictorian for the first group of women to graduate from the McGill Arts faculty. But prior to the commencement ceremony her address was censored by the principal of the university. She included the censored remarks in her delivered version nevertheless, calling for admission of women to the Faculty of Medicine. This apparent outrage brought cries of "Never!" and "Shame!" from some of the medical students present.*

Among the obstacles which women had to overcome were medical educators with serious doubts about the readiness of the community to accept female physicians. William Osler, an eminent physician of the late nineteenth and early twentieth centuries whom many consider to be the father of modern internal medicine, dealt with this "problem" in his presidential address to the Canadian Medical Association, at a time when he was working at the Montreal General Hospital:

It is useless manufacturing articles for which there is no market, and in Canada the people have not yet reached the condition in which the lady doctor finds a suitable environment. Look at the facts as they are, even the larger cities can only support one or two; in fact, Quebec and Montreal have none, and in the smaller town and villages of this country, she would starve.[16]

During the decade after Osler's speech, a few women did come to practise medicine in the province of Quebec, but not because of any benevolence or openmindedness on the part of McGill. Around 1890, just after an initiative to get women into McGill had failed, a rival school, Bishop's University, started to admit women and eventually graduated two. This enlightened policy was cut short in 1900, however, when the Montreal General Hospital amended its bylaws to preclude the training of women medical students on its wards, thereby depriving the women of Bishop's of their main source of clinical experience. Women were finally admitted at McGill in 1918, when most prospective male physicians were off at war.

Things have improved somewhat since that unbelievable era; eighteen of my classmates were women — about thirteen per cent of the class. This was in line with proportions elsewhere; the odd school admitted more women, some less.

Most universities get around the shortage of women in their

classes by citing the relatively small number applying. Although there is some truth in this, many women do not apply either because they are actively discouraged from doing so, or because of what they have heard about the experiences of women medical students.

If a woman is able to transcend the prejudice of her family, her community and her medical school admissions committee and actually makes it into medical school, she must then contend with the attitudes of her teachers and classmates. Admissions committees erroneously assume that many female physicians do not practise.[17] The indignities of the admission interview (how many children will she have? when and what sort of person will she marry?) are followed in due course by the indignities of the lecture theatre and the hospital. These can include slides of naked women interposed between pictures of pathology specimens by the lecturer as a "joke", inadequate changing facilities, and a great deal of condescension and discrimination by male members of her class.[18]

Sometimes the oppression of women in medical school is directed specifically towards their sexuality. The woman is stereotyped as either too attractive to be a physician or, contrarily, as a "horse-faced, flat-chested female in supphose who sublimates her sex starvation in a passionate embrace of *The New England Journal of Medicine*."[19]

Not all nations have made it as difficult as Canada and the United States for a woman who wants to be a physician. Women have outnumbered men in Eastern European medical schools for a long time. The trend in North America, at long last, seems to be to increase significantly the proportion of new physicians who are women; few would suggest that this is not an improvement. The indignities that women continue to experience may be, as Howard Spiro, a gastroenterologist at Yale University Medical School, has suggested, a "cultural lag" which will pass in time.[20] In the last few years there have been such hopeful signs as the willingness of medical students, men included, to confront faculty members who act in a sexist manner in class towards women students or patients.

Showing the way: the Flexner report

Medical school has not always been the preserve of the privileged; gaining admission was not always so difficult. Around the turn of the century, for example, "proprietary" medical schools flourished, in business principally to earn a profit and advertising shamelessly for students (one offering a free trip to Europe for anyone who completed three years of its programme). Much of the momentum for today's admissions policies comes from a report, *Medical Education in the United States and Canada*, that was written three-quarters of a century ago in response to this situation.[21] The report, produced by Abraham Flexner under the sponsorship of the Carnegie Foundation, and based on Flexner's visits to assess the standards of education at every medical school in the two countries, is generally regarded as one of the most important milestones in the development of North American medical education.

Before the Flexner report, medical education standards had been uneven at best and Flexner is usually given credit for raising them. The curricula in the proprietary schools were often rather informal. As medical knowledge expanded and physicians were put in the position, for the first time, of being able to do something of therapeutic benefit for their patients, it became a matter of some concern that they know what they were doing.* After publication of the report, many medical schools closed their doors. Some were schools sponsored by universities that lacked, in Flexner's view, the resources to support them.[22] Others were the "proprietary" medical schools (although it should be noted that a trend to close proprietary schools was already underway when Flexner wrote his report).

Using the Johns Hopkins Medical School as a model, Flexner determined that all students should have a solid foundation of basic scientific knowledge (not the same thing as clinical competence).[23] From a largely functional programme that was supposed to teach students how to treat the sick (and no more), Flexner pushed for a programme that "laid the scientific foundations for medical practice", an approach that has prevailed to this day and has legitimized the growth of an elite medicine — and a medical elite.

What was really at stake in Flexner's day was the role of physicians in society. At that time there was no consistent relationship between universities and medical schools and medical practice in the United States. In particular, the apprenticeship system that had characterized the early development of American medicine was in deadly competition with the medical schools, and had been for over a century. Pennsylvania, Harvard and Yale considered the physicians they trained superior to the products of the traditional educational model, and wanted their "boys" to gain the recognition they deserved. This was not easily arranged, however, because their practice of medicine was not substantially different from anyone else's. Rosemary Stevens, author of *American Medicine and the Public Interest*, writes:

Attempted distinctions between one doctor and another had to be moulded out of the educational backgrounds instead of functional differences — that is between those trained wholly by domestic apprenticeship and the small but influential group of practitioners who, by the outbreak of the revolutionary war, were receiving some kind of university education.[24]

This situation persisted despite the best endeavours of two organizations, the American Medical Association and the Association of American Medical Colleges, set up to put a professional autocracy in a position of "leadership" in American medicine.

The proprietary medical schools were an outgrowth of the apprenticeship system and, as Stevens observes, filled an important social role, at least in the nineteenth century, by providing medical care to groups, such as pioneers, who would otherwise have had none.[25] In spite of their contribution, the ever-increasing numbers of proprietary school graduates were seen by the university-trained physicians as a threat and, certainly, as an impediment to those doctors ever obtaining the status in society they desired. Nor were they likely to acquire this status when their professional title was shared with others whom they regarded as "charlatans" and, with some justification, as vestiges of the feudal era.

Putting them in historical context, proprietary schools represented a stage in American development when capital was more dispersed and free enterprise more free. The movement from apprenticeship to proprietary to university medical education was similar to processes occurring elsewhere in society: the shift, for instance, from the slave-based economy of the south and the relative free enterprise of the north (hence apprenticeship and proprietary schools) to monopoly capital (hence Big Medicine, hospital-based, with a national elite). Flexner's report was written nearly half a century after the landowner class had been routed in the Civil War by the capitalists from the north. Monopoly capital was coming into its own, as Flexner (who worked for the Rockefeller Foundation as well as for the Carnegie) knew as well as anyone. Indeed, it was extravagant funding by the big foundations that allowed the established medical schools, over the thirty years following the report, to become the powers they now are in American medicine.[26]

The report itself, though purportedly offering a disinterested evaluation of the quality of the facilities and educational programmes of the various medical schools, was full of social commentary, particularly in the introduction by Henry S. Pritchett, President of the Carnegie Foundation:

[T]he existence of many of these unnecessary and inadequate schools has been defended by the argument that a poor medical school is justified in the interest of a poor boy. It is clear that the poor boy has no right to go into any profession for which he is not willing to obtain proper preparation...

[P]rogress for the future would seem to require a very much smaller number of medical schools, better equipped and better conducted than our schools as a rule now are; and the needs of the public would require that we have fewer physicians graduated each year, but that these should be better educated and better trained.[27]

Which interests of the public, we may ask, would be better served by having fewer physicians? Especially when today, there is a shortage of medical practitioners of *any* quality for many communities.[28] But even if shortages did not exist, is it possible to imagine there being too many physicians? Pritchett apparently thought so:

In a society consituted as are our modern states, *the interests of the social order* will be served best when the number of men entering a given profession reaches and does not exceed a certain ratio. For example, in law and medicine, one sees best in a small village the situation created by the over-production of inadequately trained men. In a town of two thousand people, one will find in most states from five to eight physicians where two well-trained men could do the work efficiently *and make a competent livelihood.* When, however, six or eight physicians seek to gain a living in a town which can support only two, the whole plane of professional conduct is lowered in the struggle which ensues, each man becomes intent upon his own practice, public health and sanitation are neglected, and the ideals and standards of the profession tend to demoralization.[29]

Some of Flexner's own arguments lacked substance. For example, he cited towns of two hundred or fewer inhabitants with two or more physicians as evidence that there were too many practitioners,[30] forgetting or ignoring the possibility that such medical practices attract patients from rural areas. He concluded: "The country needs fewer and better doctors . . . [and] the way to get them better is to produce fewer."[31]

While much of what Flexner said about medical schools was true, often devastatingly so, an important consequence of his report was that fewer physicians went into practice in the United States. Clearly, there were enough physicians to serve the well-to-do, as there would always be. But the cutback in the number of physicians graduating each year led to a much-heralded physician shortage, one that is still being combatted, mostly through the importation of medical school graduates from overseas. If all of Flexner's recommendations had been followed and even more medical schools closed, the situation would now be even worse. He contended that a state or province without a medical school could always attract physicians from somewhere else.[32] If, for instance, Dalhousie University in Halifax had followed his advice[33] and closed what was, until recently, the only medical school in Atlantic Canada, there almost certainly would have been grave shortages of practitioners because, even today, most medical schools favour native sons. They do this on the reasonable assumption that if those schools do not provide doctors to their native provinces or states, no one else is going to do so.

While there were very good reasons for closing some of the atrocious medical schools that existed at the turn of the century, certain people benefited from the closures. The business community stood to benefit in at least three ways. First, it could be assured of a reasonable standard of medical care (decreasing the number of practitioners would not limit the access of the well-to-do). Secondly, businessmen's children pursuing medical careers were to be guaranteed a higher social standing. Finally, the concentration of medical education in hospitals was, in a number of ways, good for business.*

On the other hand, while the social and economic status of the medical profession was elevated, the "poor boy" was deprived of his chance to become a physician. "A mass of unprepared youth" was no longer "drawn out of industrial occupations into the study of medicine."[34] The quality of medical care may have improved but its accessibility was reduced.[35] Flexner, who was at least as concerned with limiting the number of physicians as he was with improving care, was apparently not bothered by such considerations.

Notes

page 15: In 1976, 42,155 students submitted 372,282 applications in competition for 15,774 positions in American medical schools. Thus has the market become much tighter: in 1962, 15,847 students submitted 59,054 applications for 8959 positions. (See "Medical Education in the United States", *Journal of the American Medical Association* 238 [1977]: 2770.)

page 17: Amongst applicants to Canadian medical schools in 1968, 37.2 per cent had fathers who had attended university, while at the same time less than ten per cent of the total population aged 40 to 69 had attended university. (See R.N. Jones, D.G. Fish, "Social characteristics of applicants to Canadian medical schools", *Journal of Medical Education* 45 [1970]: 918-928.)

page 18a: It is important to note that the introduction of larger numbers of people from the lower echelons of society is unlikely to make the medical profession any less conservative or more socially conscious. What data exist suggest that, if anything, the contrary may be true when no other aspects of the selection process are altered. (See J. Colombotos, "Social origins and the ideology of physicians: a study of the effects of early socialization", *Journal of Health and Social Behaviour* 10 [1969]: 16-29.)

18b: The case of *The Regents of the University of California v. Allan Bakke* was considered by many to be among the most important matters to come before the United States Supreme Court since World War Two. These are two aspects of the case that are particularly relevant to the present inquiry. The first is that although "affirmative action" programmes have affected large numbers of people in many productive sectors, it is in relation to medical school admissions, which concern relatively few, that the monumental court battle came (and attracted so much attention). The second aspect is the rationalization provided by supporters of affirmative action. Ronald Dworkin, Professor of Jurisprudence at Oxford University, who has taught at Yale and New York University Law Schools, is himself a supporter of "affirmative action" in medical schools. He is probably speaking for much of the liberal establishment when he argues that "America will continue to be pervaded by racial divisions as long as the most lucrative, satisfying and important careers remain the prerogative of the members of the white race, while others feel themselves systematically excluded from a professional and social elite." (See "Why Bakke has no case", *New York Review of Books* 24, no.18 [Nov. 10, 1977]: 11-15.) What is thus revealed is the objective of some minority admission proponents to generalize the myth that anyone can make it in America!

page 19: Why would the admissions committee have felt obliged to "crack down" on left-wing political activists? Were its members defending their own class interests? There is considerable doubt that middle-class medical students, even when turned on politically, could represent any serious threat to the established order (although this may not have been apparent). A more likely explanation is that having such people around made life more complicated — they were troublesome. It made administrative sense to keep them out.

page 20: One of the major obstacles to the admission of women seems to have been the problem of having mixed facilities: university authorities were particularly concerned about the prospect of men and women dissecting cadavers side by side.

page 22: It was not until this century that the physician-patient encounter stood a better than even chance of benefitting the patient.

page 25: This will be discussed in chapter six.

2

Call Me "Doctor"

Medical School and the Socialization Process

For most medical students, a remarkable and important transformation occurs from the time they enter medical school to the time they leave. At first, medical education is a little frightening. Typical students arrive at initial classes full of insecurity, unsure of how they ought to relate to those around them, believing there is more work to cover than time to do it in. They hold some vague fear of failure and are convinced that their classmates are better equipped to deal with it all than they themselves are.

Nothing happens right away to alleviate these anxieties. If anything, the behaviour of classmates seems to reinforce them. Because of this, the students readily accede to certain games and rituals performed by the class as a whole. These pastimes consume a great deal of energy and turn them away from more "worldly" concerns. They become immersed in the culture, environment and lifestyle of the school. They slowly lose their initial identity and become redefined by the new situation.

Medical students have to look for something to hang on to. And that something is provided: their new identity as "doctor", which becomes increasingly important as the medical years progress. So, by the time they finish medical school and as graduates are officially entitled in fact to be called Doctor (a title which, as we shall see, students actually acquire much earlier in the process), those unsure novices have gained a new professional identity that helps to define from then on their relationships with patients, other doctors and other medical support staff. It is during these years that the future doctors develop and then nurture their professional self-image.*

This process of socialization into a set role is influenced by a number of forces: the curriculum students face; the sense of competition aroused; the games and rituals they are drawn into; a remarkable and frequently pathological compulsion to work; a discouragement of an active political or critical role; and, finally, the students' own expectations of what their role should be and the resultant need to assume an identity that seems to offer the key to opening (medical) doors.

This chapter explores these forces which, operating in medical school, help to make doctors what they are.

Working hard: the medical mystique
Registration and full speed ahead

First-year medicine at McGill University does not begin with a whimper, except perhaps on the part of some students. In my own case, I suppose I might now be a lawyer — if it had not been for the cadaver.

For some time before registration, I had been vacillating between entering medicine and law. I had not been particularly enthusiastic about the prospect of signing up for either programme and had avoided making a firm commitment one way or the other. Advice didn't seem to help: one surgeon I knew told me, "Look upon it as just another year of college in which you are going to study medicine, as opposed to any other discipline. Even if you change your mind later on, the knowledge can never hurt you."

As the fateful day approached, I realized I had to make a decision. Wavering until the last minute, I finally made my choice and went off to register at the Faculty of Law. Afterwards, I went over to the medical school to let the administrators there know I was not coming. To my horror, I was shown into the office of the Associate Dean in charge of students' affairs and found myself forced to explain why I was dropping out. Unfortunately, my reasons at that point were neither immutable nor very well formulated. And, compounding my awkwardness in the situation was the guilt I felt at not having notified the medical school sooner; medical classes had begun the previous day.

"Well, what brings you here?" the Associate Dean asked with an understanding smile.

"I'm not sure I want to be a doctor," I hedged.

His eyebrows arched ever so slightly. "Have you been considering doing something else?"

"Uh, I've been thinking about law." I was playing my cards close to my chest — too close, as it turned out.

"When do you have to let them know?"

"Classes start Monday. Orientation is tomorrow."

He saw his opening and exploited it ruthlessly, smiling once again. "Well, then, why don't you go to medical classes for the rest of the week and then decide?"

Since I had not managed to tell him that I was already registered in law, I could hardly reject such a reasonable recommendation. Little did I realize that the Associate Dean had just sealed my fate. He sent me away with some homily about how it is just those students who have always been certain that they want to study medicine who most frequently have problems adjusting to medical school. I wandered over to the anatomy dissecting room where, in short order, I was swept off my feet.

It was a large rectangular room dominated by the dissecting tables. The tables held more than thirty cadavers and around them were gathered some hundred and thirty students in long white coats. I checked the list at the front of the room, quickly found my allocated position and met my three dissecting partners (Shamis, Shane and Shelbourne — I got to know the people in my class whose names began with "S" very well) and proceeded to look inside a human body for the first time. When I left that class there was really little doubt in my mind that I would return.

A few things happened to me all at once that have relevance to the experience of most medical students. First of all, I was impressed: that very first day I was confronted with a vast body of knowledge that seemed truly significant and more important than any other studies I could possibly undertake. I was humbled by the seeming infinitude of medical knowledge and by my classmates who seemed to know more of it than I did. Unlike me, they had already boned up on the pectoral muscles and surrounding structures, the day's assignment. In contrast, I felt inadequate. I was also ashamed that I had almost bypassed the opportunity to learn of such profound phenomena as the insertion of the pectoral muscles into the rib cage. In short, I had taken my place on a veritable assembly line of learning and it was obviously going to be necessary to scramble in order to keep up. Finally, I was given a first taste of a soon-to-be-realized professional role, into which I would grow (between Shane and Shelbourne) until the day of my graduation. I had found my niche.

Busy bodies: doc around the clock

Students, especially in the early stages, spend extraordinarily long hours at study without any assurance that they have mastered what is necessary. I remember well the trauma of those first days. At least some of my study time each day was wasted envisioning scenarios of my impending failure.

Most (although not all) medical students study and study and study, day in and day out. Spending so much time at this leaves that much less for everything else.* From this simple observation three questions arise. Is the time spent appropriate to what must be learned for the examinations? Is the subject matter that requires all this time as important for medical practice as the time devoted to it would suggest? What is the effect upon the student of spending so much time studying?

The time that most students spend studying far exceeds the time required merely to pass examinations. A number of students in my class were able to do well in the examinations on basic science subjects although they studied comparatively little. This was not because they were particularly brilliant but because they selectively studied the material they anticipated would appear on the examinations (in the next chapter there is more on techniques for passing examinations and otherwise acquiring knowledge). Many lose their perspective, however, when anatomy and histology replace biology and physics. Rather than approaching these subjects as simply more courses to be passed, they come to regard them as fields to be mastered. Most sport large, comprehensive textbooks, which cannot possibly be learned in a year, but which the students feel obliged to attack.

There is a popular myth that students who do not learn everything they can in medical school will not make good physicians. I remember seeing a film many years ago in which a student fell asleep during a lecture and his "sin" came back to haunt him: he subsequently committed an error that put a patient's life in jeopardy. In fact, however, there is growing recognition that much of what is taught in basic science courses is irrelevant to most medical practice.[1] All medical students are aware of this and there has been much agitation for change. In recent years most medical schools have reduced the portions of their curricula devoted to basic science.[2]

If students have been involved in extracurricular activities as undergraduates, they rapidly dissociate themselves from the friendships and activities of premedical days: no more debating, no more work on the student newspaper, no more work for the film society, no more political activism. I know that when I started first year, I was warned that I could hardly expect to keep up my own outside interests and pass (advice I now know to be quite inaccurate). Most students accept as axiomatic that they will have to leave their own interests behind them at the medical school door.*

The tendency to study excessively is clearly related to largely irrational anxieties about academic performance. One survey at McGill showed that 18.3 per cent of medical students sought help for emotional problems which, in most cases, were attributed to the process of medical education itself.[3] As F. L. McGuire has observed in his "Psycho-social studies of medical students":

[The medical student] is anxious while in pre-med training, wondering if he will be able to meet the competition and achieve high enough grades; he is anxious when he applies, feeling that his whole future is about to be decided in a few short weeks or months; and he is anxious when he begins his training. He displays a variety of anxieties during the next four years, and except for a certain amount of short-lived relief when he receives his diploma, he is still anxious when he graduates.[4]

One of my classmates arrived at the laboratory at six in the morning on his days off: an example, though extreme, of the conscientiousness of class members. Almost every student spent long hours absorbing knowledge and, because of a lack of real clinical exposure early on, or perhaps because of the distorted or confusing expectations of teachers, it was difficult to tell what was necessary for the proper practice of medicine and what was unnecessary even for the examinations.*

In *Escape from Freedom*, Erich Fromm analyzed the development of the Protestant work ethic in the face of the rise of capitalism during the Reformation:

The compulsion to unceasing effort and work was far from being in contradiction to a basic conviction of men's powerlessness; rather was it the psychological result. Effort and work in this sense assumed an entirely irrational character. They were not to change fate since this was predetermined by God, regardless of any effort on the part of the individual. They served only as a means of forecasting the predetermined fate; while at the same time frantic effort was a reassurance against an otherwise unbearable feeling of powerlessness.[5]

Similarly, students are confronted with a situation in which they feel powerlessness, insecurity and inadequacy. Their reaction is to submit before institutional authority and engage in compulsive work. While no religious doctrine is used to justify this behaviour, anxious students do, in a sense, undertake this activity to "predict their fate".

But in fact fewer students are failed today by medical schools than ever before. In the 1976-77 academic year, less than one per cent of first year students in American medical schools were obliged to withdraw for academic reasons, and another two per cent had to repeat the year.[6] In my class, given that perhaps five members would fail their first year (in fact, four did so, and all were subsequently readmitted to McGill or to other medical schools), very few members should have been troubled with fears of being Struck Down. Nonétheless, most of my classmates expressed the belief at one time or another that they might fail; some talked of little else all year, and this was even true of some of the best students. At the University of Toronto a recent survey of first-year medical students showed that the three major sources of stress reported by students were "entering the final examination in an important course", "fear of inability to master the course material" and "fear of getting bad grades".[7]

Who was responsible for the excessive fear of failure? The medical school was partly to blame. Professors relished being able to warn their classes that they could fail. However, such threats could have been ignored, as they deserved to be. That they were not is an indication of what being in medical school meant to the students. One reason for fear of failure comes from the enticements of the profession itself: the job security, community respect and status, the economic returns and the gratifying and stimulating work.

The fear of failing in medical school is, for many, the fear of having to face once again those unbearable pressures of modern society from which entry into school was to have been an escape. It is this desire to escape that propels so many into the medical school application game. It is the sense of powerlessness in society that is responsible for much of the irrational activity of students, both before and after they enter their training.

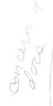

The compulsion to work of medical students reflects more than a need to escape the pressures of life. It comes partly from the emphasis on basic scientific knowledge (encouraged by Abraham Flexner), as opposed to clinical competence, as the foundation of medical learning. It represents also an attempt by the students to immerse themselves in and become part of something big and powerful. They readily submerge in a professional role and internalize the compulsion to work. The latter becomes integral, in fact, to their burgeoning professional identity, and it drives them as no external authority could.*

These processes play an important role in the education of the physician at every stage. All medical students are affected by them in some degree, and so is the entire medical profession.

After graduation, when physicians-in-training go to work in a hospital as house officers — a category that includes both interns and residents — the going gets even rougher as the hours of labour increase yet again. There has been a great deal of literature on this subject. An anonymous "Doctor X", in a book called *Intern*, has written a journal describing his internship.[8] One cannot help but be moved, when reading this document, by the continual exhaustion of the man. William Nolan, author of *The Making of a Surgeon,* has recorded the hardships that being a physician-in-training brings to married life.[9] David Bell, in *A Time to be Born,* has written about the trying work schedule of a resident in pediatrics.[10] Another physician, Robin Cook, has written *Year of the Intern* primarily to expose the extent to which house officers are overworked. In it he describes the effects that overwork has upon them both as people and as physicians.[11]

Notwithstanding these poignant memoirs, house officers are not working as hard today as they once did. Today, the average house officer in most North American hospitals spends one night in every three on duty. There are exceptions: surgical house staff tends to work more often than this, staff in psychiatry less often. This is a far cry from the horrors of not too many years ago when physicians-in-training lived in the hospital (residents were really residents) and only occasionally had time off. Now, at least in Los Angeles, residents often take advantage of the less rigorous on-call schedule to "moonlight" for extra money.

During training, my on-call schedule ranged from one night in two to one in five. The contract we had signed called for one night in four, but this was rarely observed. The general medical wards usually worked interns two nights of every five, and the general surgical floors usually slated them for duty every second night. Other rotations were less gruelling.

Most nights on call weren't too bad, but sorrows really did come in battalions. The sleepless night, when it occurred, was followed by a full day on duty during which it was necessary to carry on normally, in spite of being sleep-deprived. As Dr. Cook suggests, such fatigue can hamper the ability of the physician-in-training to make decisions that, at least occasionally, affect the well-being of others:

[T]he intern gropes inside himself and makes arbitrary decisions, depending on how tired he is, whether it is morning or night, whether he is in love or lonely. And then he tries to forget them, which is easy if he is tired; and, because he's always tired, he always forgets — except that later the memory may surface from his unconscious. Angry and uncertain, he has once more been tested and found unprepared.[12]

House officers can usually summon their resources, regardless of how tired they are, to make decisions in an emergency situation. However, there is no doubt in my mind that patient care sometimes suffered when my colleagues and I were functioning well below our potential because of exhaustion.

Another consequence of a murderous work schedule is that resident physicians tend to relate less to patients as people than as problems to be dealt with impersonally. As "Doctor X" puts it:

With the kind of patient flow that we've been having, which has been heavy almost to the point of the ridiculous, and with the rarity of any kind of personal contact with most of them, it is just amazingly easy to fall into the trap that always made me so mad in medical school of regarding the patient, quite sincerely, as a leg, or a shoulder, or a gall bladder.[13]

Dr. Cook notes that he came to look at patients the same way during his internship: "Over the months my attitude toward (the patient) had changed. Each case became an organ, a specific disease, or a procedure."[14]

The overwork of the house officers (who cannot help but feel, at least at times, that they are being exploited) exacerbates their inability to relate humanely to their work and thereby increases their alienation from patients. Cook touches on this as well:

I'm being exploited under the guise of learning, the psychological burden is too heavy . . . Eventually you reach a point where you don't give a damn. Sometimes, after getting called on a cardiac arrest in the middle of the night, I suddenly realize that I wish the guy would die so I could go back to bed. I mean that's how tired and pissed off I get.[15]

While this doctor is clearly stressed by his fatigue, the cause of alienation is more than this. In fact, as we shall see, very few doctors can relate to their patients in a humane and sensitive way under the given conditions and structure of medical work today.

Besides its effects on patient care, hard work has an impact on a house doctor's relationship to the world outside the hospital, just as it does on a student's. On one level, social life can be severely compromised; try as I did, I gradually lost touch with most of my non-medical friends while I was in training, so different was my work schedule from theirs. The only option available in such a situation is to relate to hospital people; this cannot but reinforce the overwhelming presence of the hospital and of medicine in the life of the young man or woman in white.

Total involvement in hospital work contributes to house officers' dependence upon the hospital and upon the familiar, structured training programmes, making it unlikely that they will strike out in new directions once they have finished. After all, how much in the way of spontaneity can we expect from newly-trained specialists who have done little but work hard at pursuing their certificate for eight years or more? Their creativity is bound to have diminished in that near-decade of conformity and even if the creativity is still there, their confidence in their ability to act originally will have disappeared.

Another effect of the endless hard work of the house officer, according to some analyses, is the development of a "Now I'm going to get mine" attitude. Cook states it bluntly.

About half the time since third-year medical school has been spent in pursuit of the useless and the arbitrary, which are justified by the diaphanous explanation that they are a necessary part of being a medical student or intern and becoming a doctor. Bullshit. This sort of thing is simply a hazing and harassment, a kind of initiation rite into the American Medical Association. The system works, too; God, how it works! Behold the medical profession, brainwashed, narrowly programmed, right wing in its politics, and fully dedicated to the pursuit of money . . .

I felt I had done my time. . . . Medical practice was at last within sight. As I walked down the OR corridor, I wondered whether to buy a Mercedes or a Porsche. [16]

In all fairness, it should be said that not all graduating physicians are cynical or even politically conservative. In fact, I don't think that the members of my class could be described as any more conservative than any comparable group of students in any other professional faculty. Many would probably develop more conservative ideas as they went along (indeed, some had already begun to do so) but that is what generally happens to people as they become increasingly affluent.

But is the compulsion towards hard work some kind of conspiracy against the trainee? I think not; hospitals have been run that way for as long as any of the physicians who are in practice can remember, and it would be difficult for many to imagine things being substantially different. Furthermore, although many physicians-in-training protest regularly about how hard they have to work, most throw themselves into their work with considerable gusto — frequently more than is required. The few times I heard anyone point out that the clause in our contract obliging us to work no more than one night in four was not being respected, the majority of house officers present expressed the view that we were better off working more nights, because we learned more that way.

Even many of the physician-authors who have criticized their overwork tend to be self-contradictory. They all describe some high and poignant moments in the midst of their exhausting ordeal, moments they seem to cherish. With the exception of Cook all seem inclined, in the balance, to accept the hardship for the fine feelings it arouses.

Another reason why resident physicians are so accepting of

their ordeal, and why physicians in practice look back on their internships as the high point of their training, is that the ritual of overwork allows them to submerge almost totally in the medical environment, to the exclusion of most other concerns. The moments that I felt best about my work as an intern usually came in the middle of the night when, as the city and most of the hospital slept, I rushed down some dark corridor towards some ailing person. There is a tendency (to which I succumbed) to say to yourself: "Aren't I great? Look what I am doing to help other people."

As a mechanism of escape, at least some of the hard work of interns is welcomed by them, as it was in the preclinical years. The only differences are that the internal compulsion to work has strengthened over the years, and that it is now buttressed by the external authority of their employer cum educator, the hospital.

Anatomy of a curriculum

Neither the medical school nor its curriculum is an undifferentiated entity. A medical school consists of a number of remarkably independent academic departments, each with its own set of priorities, attitudes, orientations and objectives, loosely co-ordinated by the Office of the Dean. The departments differ as widely in their relative influence over priorities and programmes in the school as they do in their internal affairs. And, it seems, it is often the power relationships between departments, rather than the actual needs of the community or students, that determines the emphasis placed on subjects in the curriculum.

The medical course I experienced at McGill was a typical one in many respects. Its four-year duration was divided into two major phases: the *basic science* or *preclinical* part, involving subjects such as anatomy, biochemistry, pathology and microbiology; and the *clinical* part, with studies in areas such as internal medicine, surgery, gynecology and psychiatry. The preclinical studies, largely limited to classroom and laboratory work, occupy the first year and a half of the programme.

At McGill, the basic science departments (those charged with teaching most of the first two years of the medical course) were anatomy, biochemistry, physiology, history of medicine, pathology, microbiology, epidemiology and pharmacology. The most powerful of these departments was anatomy. The anatomists were responsible for teaching two courses in the first year: gross anatomy and histology (the study of tissues). These were Heavy Courses for the students, especially gross anatomy (or, as we called it, just plain "anatomy"). Far more hours were devoted to the teaching of anatomy in first year than to any other subject.

The anatomy course was taught by the traditional method: dissection of cadavers. This is not a particularly efficient way of delivering the essentials to the student, who can pick them up just as well and much more quickly when predissected specimens, called prosections, are used.[17] It is, however, as I found on the first day of my medical education, a most effective way of making students concentrate on the study of anatomy.

McGill taught anatomy very well. At each sitting of United States National Board of Medical Examiners examinations, which permitted comparison of students' knowledge in different medical schools throughout North America, McGill students ranked at or near the top in anatomy. That was not a particularly wondrous achievement; we were taught twice as many hours of anatomy as in the average medical school.*

Other departments had much smaller time allocations. The Department of Epidemiology delivered a course on the prevalence, distribution and prevention of disease, with comparatively little time devoted to it. Furthermore, the hours allotted were often stuck on at the end of a long session of lectures in more "important" courses like pathology, so many students went off to study (or to sleep) during epidemiology lectures. Most students recognized that the material being covered in epidemiology had considerable relevance to their ultimate practice of medicine, but given their perspective as students, the course itself was not looked upon as important, surprising as that may seem. For one thing, epidemiology had a reputation for never failing anyone, while anatomy, with a reputation for being cold-blooded, seemed to require much more attention to get a pass; all it took to be faced with an extra summer's work in the laboratory was failure to identify a sufficient proportion of labelled body parts during a twenty minute tour through a room full of cadavers. Every member of the class spent countless nights pouring over lecture notes, texts and anatomical atlases, and many weekend days in the laboratory reviewing specimens. The epidemiology course got the once-over treatment the night before the examination, from those students who studied it at all.*

There is no consensus among medical educators as to precisely how many hours ought to be devoted to each subject in the medical school curriculum. Those who have given any thought to the problem, however, generally agree that anatomy is relatively less important than it once was, and that epidemiology and related subjects (preventive medicine and public health) are not sufficiently emphasized. In their published objectives, many medical schools indicate that they favour such a reorientation. Unfortunately, they usually do not practise what they preach.

There was a time when the dissection of the cadaver constituted the major part of a physician's education. Not too many years ago, North American medical students had to rob graves to obtain bodies for the dissecting tables.* For a long time there was not much more than anatomy to be taught, since the physician had so little to offer his patients that was likely to be of much benefit therapeutically. The bulk of the physician's skill was the ability to diagnose and all this amounted to was the capacity to elicit symptoms, to examine the patient carefully, and to draw limited conclusions from the synthesis of this data.

Biochemistry, pathology and microbiology came into their own at the turn of the century. Pharmacology took off when antibiotics were introduced during the Second World War. Immunology as a significant entity in the curriculum is even newer and in many schools does not yet constitute a separate course. The totality of knowledge in these disciplines is said to be doubling every five to ten years! Few would make such a claim for gross anatomy, where nothing new under the skin has transpired for years. It is logical that as these newer disciplines come to play an ever more important role in the scientific basis of medical practice, a greater proportion of the student's time should be ceded to them by the anatomists.

But this had still not happened at McGill by the time I finished medical school. Why not? The answer is simple enough: the anatomy course remained dominant because the anatomy department itself was so powerful. The chairman of the department was an internationally-renowned researcher, one of the most respected men in his field. In that sense, he was a distinct credit to the university and its medical school. He was able to attract considerable funding for research. He enhanced the school's reputation. He also believed that the anatomy course was important and its stature should not be diminished. He held considerable sway over the deliberations of the curriculum committee; the university could not afford to offend him and run the risk of losing him, along with his prestige and his research money.

There were, of course, other departments competing successfully for power alongside anatomy. Recently, for instance, the Department of Pharmacology had come into ascendance in curriculum planning, after hiring as a head its own "internationally-renowned" scientist, who in turn attracted other "first-rate" researchers.

There are several reasons why departments vie for time in the medical school curriculum. One reason is that the more hours available to them for teaching, the better able they are to demonstrate their interest and status in educating medical students and from that enable themselves to defend their important secondary objective:

the "pursuit of truth" through research. In addition there is the self-esteem of teachers; some consider it a personal as well as professional affront to have their course time slashed in favour of another department. There is, as well, a less petty aspect to self-esteem: the belief of a scientist in his or her discipline. As one biochemistry professor put it, "No one wants to see a downgrading of the material he has devoted his life to. If the discipline is downgraded, so is your self-esteem." Increasing government subsidization of medical education, along with unstable research funding, have made many departments anxious to be seen as making an important contribution to the teaching of medical students. Funding is not yet proportional to hours taught, but many departments have seen the writing on the wall and, having no shortage of teachers available to occupy the classroom, have acted accordingly.

Other schools operate much the same way as McGill. In general, established medical schools tend more to stress the traditional basic sciences while newer ones, having started afresh, with fewer vested interests to consider, are oriented more to social and preventive medicine. Even in these schools, however, there is frequently a slip towards the priorities of the older institutions. In order to establish "names" for themselves, they try to attract superstar researchers, with predictable consequences for the curriculum.*

The power of a department is consistently a function of its ability to contribute to the prevailing emphasis of the faculty. If the dominant ideology is scholarship (research), then the distinguished researcher will call the shots. If areas such as public health, community medicine, or psycho-social aspects of medicine are emphasized, then teachers who excel at those will be most influential. Just as anatomists do not want to see their discipline diminished, so too will other teachers defend the interests of their discipline when its standing is threatened. Those Flexnerian "scientific foundations", which form the basis of much of the physician's claim to a professional role, are not a careful construct with objective validity, but an outcome of power struggles in the medical school for a larger share of the student's time. The anatomy of the curriculum was no more an objective reality in Flexner's day than it is now. Then, too, it was the triumph of some vested interests (the medical establishment) over others (the proprietary schools).

But in no real sense can the allocation of time in the medical course be considered a synthesis of judgements of learned, disinterested scholars in the field of medical education. It is more a reflection of the power structure of the medical school. It becomes apparent that such an arrangement does not inevitably (or even usually) lead to a curriculum relevant to the needs of future physicians or of the society in which they will practise.

Wrestling with shadows: games and rituals

From the first day of medical school to graduation, throughout internship and long thereafter, physicians-in-training are kept busy — and it is not only with those things usually thought of as work or study. Games and rituals related to medical school and to the developing role of the professional occupy so much energy that it is not surprising there is so little time, or even need, to think about anything other than medicine.

That games, or competition, are such an established way of life in medical school is clearly related to students' obsessions with failing or doing badly. This explanation is incomplete, however, for at least two reasons. First, the fear of failing is usually far out of proportion to the real risk involved and is really only an excuse for the frantic activity that satisfies other needs. Secondly, competitiveness is not an inevitable consequence of the student situation. The opposite might even be anticipated: that students would *avoid* competitiveness to reduce tension.

It is in the anatomy laboratory, where groups of three or four students work together over a specimen, that medical students first "come out" as competitors. Inevitably, students enter the laboratory on a given day in different states of preparation. Some know a great deal about the part of the body being dissected, others little if anything. All members of a group can see just how knowledgeable they are in relation to the others — an ideal starting point for competition. Students in command of the most knowledge control a very potent commodity, theirs to distribute as they see fit. They may do so with patience and understanding, or with condescension and pained reluctance, if at all.

Encounters between students in the anatomy laboratory frequently follow the second pattern: manipulation, indifference and competition predominate, and the name of the game is *I know more than you do.*

In this game, less knowledgeable students are the invariable losers. The time will soon come when they will choose to conceal their ignorance rather than risk yet another round of embarrassment and humiliation. The "winners" of the game do not abuse their classmates in this way just to be mean. They have worked hard and, still insecure in their knowledge, may feel exploited when a student who has worked less hard pries some knowledge from them. Tension runs high in the anatomy laboratory (which might better be called the "anxiety laboratory"); students feel pressed to master a great deal of material in a very short time. Getting back at a classmate may provide a convenient outlet for frustration with work. It serves as a means to redistribute, to another classmate, the students' own anxieties about a course at the same time as bolstering their own confidence.

A related game popular amongst medical students might be called *I know something you don't know*, and it is played in the corridors and cafeterias as well as in the classrooms and laboratories. In this game, one student quizzes another about some obscure point in the full expectation that the other will not know the answer. The second competitor usually retorts with an esoteric question of his or her own. The game can go on and on, one obscure question followed by another one even more obscure. The questions are rarely, if ever, based on material students are likely to be asked about on an examination, and they are even less relevant to medical practice.

Not all students play, of course. Students who are having problems with their work or who are just not able to perform in this format are intimidated by these sessions, which they encounter every day and in which they are constantly being asked to engage.

Why is this game so popular? It certainly has no value as a learning device. But because anxiety is their usual state, students seek positive feedback about their progress, and this is seldom forthcoming from the faculty. Hence they attempt to prove themselves at the expense of their colleagues. The contests are usually inconclusive, because each competitor inevitably knows a few facts that others do not and ultimately everybody's anxiety increases; the big losers are those who are not able to compete. Several of my classmates admitted to looking up obscure facts and committing them to memory just so they would not be overwhelmed when thrust into one of these trivia quizzes.

Another favourite game — most frequently played in the library — is *I can study longer than you can*. Students who spend much less time than others at their work will often feel guilty and inadequate as a result, whether or not the work is really necessary. They frequently study late just because their classmates are doing so too, or stay on in the library even when their work is finished only because their classmates have not yet left (no doubt for the same reason). Some of my classmates lived in a university residence. They reported that when one of them went into the common room and saw that the others were not there, that student would return to his or her own room to study some more for fear of being outflanked. This behaviour, of course, did nothing to make anyone less anxious. Not all students played this game. Those who did not, however, were often haunted by self-doubt.[18]

Gamesmanship also finds its way into the classroom, where students play *Move to the front of the class*. Competitiveness in this sphere does not spring directly from the pursuit of marks. Student performance in class is rarely if ever a factor in computing grades. There is a group of students in every medical class who are inevitably and invariably in control. They pepper the professor with questions, correct any errors made and race to be first to respond to questions. Except for lectures that are entirely didactic, most degenerate into a dialogue between the professor and these few students.

If most students say nothing in class, it is not always because they have nothing to say. Many are afraid to ask a question (or to answer one) for fear of appearing foolish. The potential of the educational experience is considerably diminished for many who sit nervously through a lecture, hardly following the material, fearful that they will be singled out to answer a question.

It is not the professor they fear. Often as not they will not be seeing that particular teacher again. The fear of participating in class is the fear of being humiliated in the eyes of classmates. To appear ignorant is to become even more insecure, a feeling often enhanced by class members all too happy to lord it over colleagues with their superiority of knowledge in the thousand ways in which this can be done.*

This inability to participate in classroom discussions makes it all the harder for students to catch on and catch up; it reinforces gaps in knowledge between classmates. One should obviously not find it a major embarrassment to admit that one does not understand something. The students are relating destructively, however; as in the other instances, some students are attempting to alleviate their anxiety at the expense of others by demonstrating their own superiority.

Another very perverse game that medical students play is related to their fear of failing: *the numbers game*. Each student estimates how many are likely to fail (a particular course or the entire year) and proceeds to count heads, the object being to count oneself out of the ranks of the doomed. The rules of the game are simple enough. First identify the students who are likely to fail. Next, identify those students who will not necessarily fail, but who seem to know less than you. Add these two groups together; if their numbers exceed the expected failures, the game is won. Lastly, make it a point to express concern for the welfare of a classmate who seems to be in trouble.

Protestations of sympathy are an important part of this game. In my class, one fellow in particular was widely expected to fail. Some talked endlessly about how "poor J. isn't going to make it". Had they spent half as much time helping J. as they did bemoaning his plight he might have done much better. One could sense that some were almost relieved to see that he was having so much trouble. After all, one man so obviously marked to fail was one less who had to be beaten in the numbers game.*

Class rank is another popular game in medical school, particularly around examination time. The special forms of competition that occur at this time can be particularly destructive. Until recently, McGill posted a pass list of medical students in rank order from first to last, a practice common to many medical schools at the time. This certainly fostered competitiveness. Students were aware that they would be asked their class rank when applying for postgraduate positions. It was a cruel ploy on the part of the school: even a small difference in grade (and an even smaller difference in knowledge) could mean a great difference in class standing. Only in the most tenuous way did the ranking reflect any significant reality.

The system of absolute ranking was eventually discarded in favour of one that rated the student as being in the upper, middle, or lower third of the class. This finally gave way in my year to the system that has now become the most fashionable. Called the **pass-fail system**, it involves giving students a report card indicating only whether they have passed or failed. The reason for changing to such a system was to eliminate destructive competitiveness. It has not succeeded in achieving this, however, because it is not really a pass-fail system. Marks *are* recorded and the Dean scrutinizes them carefully when sending a letter to a hospital on behalf of an applicant for an internship. Then, without saying explicitly what the student's grades are, the Dean scrupulously makes sure the strength of endorsement reflects the recorded standing.

This game is now being played by a substantial proportion of medical schools, so intern selection committees have inevitably turned to linguistic analysis to decipher the students' grades. A member of one such committee at a hospital in California, which regularly receives large numbers of applications from students at eastern schools, reported: "We have never received a letter from Harvard that rated a student less than 'good'. They describe most of their students as 'outstandingly exceptional', 'brilliant', or something of that order. We have more or less figured out what the hierarchy of such rankings is. When the occasional fellow shows up from Harvard with a standing of 'good', we know he isn't up to scratch."

Students who want to "make it" have to perform appropriately, so the game of class rank remains an important pastime in the medical school classroom. As the prestigious internship becomes harder to come by, classroom combat becomes even fiercer. Nor does this game end with the transition to the hospital. In the latter years of medical school, the rating of students is done jointly by teachers and some residents with whom the students have been in contact on the wards of the hospital. In this setting, students are compared directly to colleagues they have been working with. For the ambitious students, it is particularly important to outshine the next person; competition can be vicious, because each student is aware that not all will make it to the promised land.

During my third-year rotation in internal medicine, I toured the wards in the company of four other students and a tutor. The tutor would ultimately decide, along with a few others, how good we were and for those of us with an interest in postgraduate training in internal medicine, his recommendations would be particularly important. Every day, as we "rounded" with our well-meaning tutor, each of us could tell just where we stood in his estimation and we became competitive in all sorts of subtle ways. The whole game became something of a joke after a while. A student whom the tutor particularly favoured was greeted each day by the others with "Good morning, Number One". One who had fallen into disfavour became known as Number Five. When rankings changed, as they occasionally did, we ceremoniously congratulated the person who had been promoted. Only occasionally did the tutor's perceptions of our relative capabilities bear much relationship to reality, and there was considerable resentment in the group that one student was able to convey to the tutor the impression of being much more skilled and knowledgeable than was actually warranted.*

Are students, then, to blame for these games? Destructive competition does serve a purpose for them, and the games would not be played if students were not attempting to benefit from them in some way. However, the medical school actively promotes competitiveness, both by creating anxiety and by repeatedly humiliating the student. Though competitiveness is often self-defeating, it is not necessarily illogical in the context of the *irrational authority* (to use Fromm's formulation) of the medical school and its curriculum. Oppressive and unhealthy interaction and competition among medical students are direct consequences of an oppressive and unhealthy environment.

The ritual of examinations

All other events in the scholastic year pale in significance next to the ever-ominous, ever-approaching spectre of examinations. Students become far more concerned with passing them than with profiting from the educational process in any meaningful way.* Exams can destroy students' careers or catapult them to a level of "achievement" that opens new doors. This they accept, although knowing that performance on an examination is not an accurate reflection of mastery of the subject matter and has almost no relation to subsequent performance as a physician.[19] It is only superficially paradoxical that students who are so concerned with examinations are often unable to confront the necessary studying efficiently and realistically.

Examinations become not a measurement but a trial by ordeal in which students who can hold their psyches together, not succumbing to physical fatigue or to intimidation, will triumph. Cynical at first, even hostile, students come in the end to believe in the merits of the process, even to express admiration for those who perform better (as if it really mattered).

At McGill, examinations were held about four times a year throughout the four years of medical school. In my class, tensions would begin to rise weeks in advance, escalating rapidly as the fateful day drew near. At some schools, examinations are held less often, but the psychological trauma is no less severe, and the effects are no less enduring.

The examination process renders students even more vulnerable to the socializing tendencies of the medical school environment. The examination serves as a rite of passage into a new identity. In his book *Deschooling Society* Ivan Illich writes:

School serves as an effective creator and sustainer of social myth because of its structure as a ritual game of graded promotions. Introduction into this gambling ritual is much more important than what or how something is taught. It is the game itself that schools, that gets into the blood and becomes a habit.[20]

Students are taught to approach medicine as a game in which they can progress by achieving a standard established by someone else. Whatever reservations they may have about the process, the ritual activity of examination-centred life overwhelms most skepticism. The notion that one's advancement to a subsequent activity should be adjudicated (and even timetabled) by the authorities of an institution is accepted by virtually all medical students. (This is so in spite of the fact that medical educators do not agree on what aspects of future competence for medical practice are being measured by the examinations.) While they may quibble about specifics of the examining process, students do not argue that the system itself be abandoned and that they be allowed to move onto a more advanced level when, say, both they themselves and their colleagues deem them ready.

So inured are the medical schools and their authorities to life organized around examinations that it is considered deviant to take time away from the pursuit of promotions to develop other interests. Premedical students who do so are suspect, their inability to follow a straight line to medical school being generally held against them. One classmate of mine took some time off from medical school at the end of second year to 'work things out'. When he returned a year later, he was obliged to submit to a psychiatric examination before being readmitted! As if it were not enough to discourage such endeavours, the student who seeks to express the spontaneity and creativity that has no outlet in the medical school is presumed to be mentally unstable.

The examination ritual, like the games medical students play, helps to promote a whole way of life. If students are kept busy enough they will not have time to think about anything else. Their experience is similar to a ride on a roller coaster: concerned with not being ejected from the seat at some unexpected turn; totally involved in the ride, its trials and thrills; feeling at once powerful yet impotent; unable to think beyond the bounds of the train itself; everything else becomes blurred, indistinct and finally irrelevant.*

The ritual of choosing electives

There is a relatively new ritual practised by students in many medical schools. It begins the day students first ask themselves: "Where should I do my elective?"

Blocks of elective time, some quite long, have been introduced into the curricula of most medical schools in North America over the last two decades. The intention, presumably, is to allow students to pursue their own interests.

This should be a happy development: is it not that opportunity to grow freely and spontaneously which has been lacking in so much of medical education? But in fact, these blocks of time are far from being such an opportunity. Students who hope to land internships or residencies in a particular field are now more or less obliged to take electives in that same specialty to ingratiate themselves with the people who can write letters of recommendation on their behalf.

Another popular method for using elective time to advantage is to do an elective in the hospital where one is applying for a postgraduate position. Particularly when the hospital is out of town, this may be the only hope of making a significant impression on the selection committee. Thus there are certain advantages to worrying long in advance about how these valuable bits of time can be most wisely invested.

Of course, not all students are so cold-blooded about the use of their elective time. Some do electives in fields that they think are important but that they will not have an opportunity to get involved in during their residencies. Thus the future general practitioner does electives in dermatology and ophthalmology. Others use their electives to escape from the pressures of the medical curriculum by going to far away places where the work won't be too hard. England and Africa are favourites, as is the Caribbean in the wintertime. Still other students use their electives to find out if they like a particular specialty or subspeciality.

The choice, then, is anything but spontaneous. Based as it is on a variety of practical considerations, it mostly accomplishes the more efficient processing of medical students along the road to ultimate careers. Actually, the 'choice' is largely illusory, since the needs that dictate the selection of a particular elective are those the students' education has generated.

Did any students use their electives to do something quite different, perhaps following more creative or alternative approaches? One member of my class did an elective in which he examined interaction in a hospital clinic. Another did an elective in the history of medicine. I did one with a provincial government working group on health care policy. There were probably a few other such electives, none of which constituted a challenge to established norms. Even if we suppose there to have been ten or twelve such different electives in a class of 135 (and I don't think there were that many), that certainly doesn't point to a great deal of spontaneous self-direction. The social and psychological contingencies of medical school are such that even if *all* time is made elective in theory (as was done at one California medical school), very few students stray from the beaten track. For the bulk of students, the electives contribute to the ritualization of progress through medical school, obliging students to plan years ahead and close many doors to open just one. Because they think it necessary to make their choices so early, students become very career-oriented.* Medical students who choose their elective on the basis of whether they want to apply to ophthalmology or to otolaryngology after they intern are hardly going to stop and ask themselves fundamental questions, either about their educational experience or about their place in society: the trees have made the forest invisible. The electives that are not really electives mesh with the career options that are not really options but predictable outcomes of a medical education.* Commenting on the "changes" in medical education, a health services researcher at UCLA told me recently, "They may have given it fins, put a hole in the roof and painted it a different colour, but it still has four wheels and an internal combustion engine.''

The internship application ritual

Early in medical school, students become aware of the difficulty of securing a 'desirable' internship. In spite of the fact that there are more positions available each year than there are graduates from medical schools in North America, many students are frustrated in their efforts to obtain jobs they really want: they have become convinced that there are only a few jobs really worthy of them. Thus there is the spectacle of 1000 students applying for 20 positions in internal medicine at a popular university hospital. And, while most are ultimately obliged to settle for less, few are willing to accept so 'little' as a community hospital.

Are the university hospitals really that much better as places to train? Other than the inferior working conditions you find in some (and certainly not all) community hospitals, there is really not that much to choose. University hospitals expose the trainee to theory; community hospitals give more in the way of practical experience. As one neurologist put it: "Those guys who intern at an academic hospital are crazy — they never get to do anything." If there is any advantage to the university hospitals, it is in the calibre of resident physicians who, in theory at least, do much of the teaching.

Whatever their real merit, the pursuit of the desired internships begins in first year, when even the students who do not have specialties in mind begin to think seriously about strategies to secure internships. Through the four years of medical school, the concern with the choice of hospital grows into an obsession that, by the end, overshadows all else.

This preoccupation blends well into the fabric of other games and rituals that keep the medical student busy. This was brought home to the members of my class with devastating clarity at the end of our third year.

On that occasion, we wrote a series of final examinations which, as usual, had us biting our nails until the last day of school. Fortunately, only one of the series was to be decisive in our year's grades; that was pharmacology. On the last day of these examinations, as we left the examination room, we were each handed a slip of paper that told us if we had passed pharmacology and, in effect, the year.

Those of us who passed (few failed) left the room with the feeling that a ton of bricks had been lifted from our shoulders. The crisis over, we proceeded into a lecture theatre where a professor jolted at least some of us by announcing that we must soon begin preparing our applications for internships.

Never more than on that day did I feel like a passive object being processed along a conveyor belt. We were not even given a moment after that examination to regain our bearings, but were instead force-marched to the next preordained stage.

What do the games and rituals add up to? They keep students involved with fairly specific concerns: their advancement through medical school, their professional self-image and particular aspects of their future professional activity. Ivan Illich says that rituals in the educational process reinforce "the myth of unending consumption".[21] Students play games and perform rituals in the belief that these devices will facilitate attainment of a particularly desirous objective, like a medical degree or a good internship. They never transcend the rituals, however, because once involved in this way, the students acquire new needs and objectives, which are functions mostly of the games being played. At each stage the play becomes more intense and, for students who entered the game in search of security, the objective becomes ever more elusive as they pursue it in a destructive milieu of increasingly structured consciousness and progressively deteriorating human relationships.

Ultimately students become defined by their objectives and can rationalize all their otherwise pointless activity in terms of it. As Illich says:

Rituals can hide from their participants even discrepancies and conflicts between a social principle and social organization. As long as an individual is not explicitly conscious of the ritual character of the process through which he was initiated to the forces which shape his cosmos, he cannot break the spell and shape a new cosmos.[22]

Social awareness, where it exists, loses priority or vanishes. Like students being processed through other professional schools, medical students must become adept in the games and rituals of their educational experience if they are to achieve their goal. In the end it is perhaps the lesson of gamesmanship that is learnt best of all.

Student activism . . . . and its failure

Every day students have to make decisions that reflect their own social outlook. Some of these decisions, such as the way they choose to relate to nurses and orderlies, are taken by the individuals involved without any particular consultation with colleagues. Others are much more public and involve taking positions on issues that have been actively discussed by members of the class.

The Student Health Organization (SHO), established with so much idealistic enthusiasm by health science students in the United States in the late sixties and funded in its endeavours by the American federal government, did not live up to expectations. It organized projects throughout the country through which students could work during their summer vacations in community health programmes aimed at the poor. Some of the participants in these programmes were fairly sophisticated politically, and hoped to use the SHO as a focus for the development of more progressive and political medical programmes. They looked beyond their projects to "a coalition of students and community activists", but in so doing, isolated themselves from any of the students who had been attracted to the programme from a less ideological point of view. This contradiction between radical objectives and liberal justifications caused the SHO to founder.[23]

Soon after, the main focus for student activism in American medical schools had become the Medical Committee for Human Rights (MCHR). This group began as an organization through which some young physicians provided money and medical assistance for the civil rights movement. At first "apolitical", it soon became "the voice of humanist medicine" and later acquired a socialist perspective. Throughout this evolution, the MCHR consisted almost entirely of health professionals and medical students; these people had considerable difficulty developing the broad coalition of workers and consumers envisioned in the later days of the SHO.[24]*

Only small numbers of students ever became active in (or even sympathetic towards) any of these organizations, for the simple reason that most students did not recognize it as being in their interest to do so. Most of those involved had been active as undergraduates in the anti-war movement and other forms of left-wing campus politics. The activist inclinations of many diminished as they progressed through medical school, and even those whose commitment did not fade faced monumental difficulties in mobilizing their colleagues.

In the few years before I entered medical school, some students at McGill had attempted to bring their social idealism to bear upon problems relating to health. Paralleling developments in the United States, they established the McGill Student Health Organization (later renamed the Montreal Student Health Organization) to work for health action in the community. These students played a major role in the establishment of a community clinic now run by the citizens of the Pointe Ste. Charles area of Montreal. In addition they held seminars intended to sensitize medical students to social issues, naming the sponsoring organization the Norman Bethune Society after the McGill surgeon who became a hero and martyr of the Chinese revolution.

In the class prior to mine, quite a few students had been close to the New Left as undergraduates. They brought their activism to medical school, organizing protests against some of the city's more oppressive health care facilities. As they became more involved in their studies, the activism of the members of that class declined precipitously, but a few retained their involvement. One of these students reports that, because of his reputation as a "troublemaker", he was advised by the head of one clinical department that he would have to "do very well" in order to pass the course he was taking in that Chief's department. Such tools for socialization can be quite effective (and not surprisingly). Those who fail to follow the carrot will usually succumb to the stick.

The faculty members did not want a repeat performance of this previous class and selected for my year students they felt would be much more conservative. A repeat performance there most certainly was not, and our teachers congratulated us *ad nauseam* for being so much more docile than our predecessors. However, they probably need not have worried. Interest in politics began to diminish at campuses around the world (including McGill) shortly after its brief flowering, partly because of the "winding down" of the war in Vietnam and partly because students began to be afflicted by economic insecurity. The medical school environment did much to encourage this process in its peculiarly vulnerable charges.

Aside from the very small numbers of students involved in the MCHR (and most medical schools lacked *any* such organization), most reformist zeal was directed towards changing the curriculum. At McGill in 1968 — the year before I entered medical school — an advisory committee on the undergraduate medical curriculum had been established to consider how the content of the medical course should evolve. A number of members of my class became quite actively involved in this committee's deliberations during our first three years. In the end, however, curriculum reform manifested the near-impossibility of effecting substantial change in medical education.

There was a clear student consensus on many of the issues being discussed by the committee. Students wanted the time devoted to anatomy diminished and clinical training introduced before the end of second year. They were also unhappy with the haphazard organization of the curriculum: different departments taught courses about the same disease and organ systems at different times and quite independently of one another. Finally, many students wanted to see more elective time in the course, so they could explore those areas of medicine that interested them most.

The students involved in the committee were quite serious about making the curriculum more palatable, efficient and flexible. They wanted to develop a curriculum more in keeping with the needs and aspirations of their colleagues, to make medical school a more satisfying place for students to be. As one class member who was active in curriculum wrote:

A student's choices will be *for himself* and will not restrict the opportunity of other students to meet their needs. However, in the long run these choices will be significant not only for the individual student, but in guiding the incorporation of elective courses into the core programme and in the establishment of new electives.[25]

Nothing that was proposed could have been interpreted as a threat to established medical practice or to the priorities of academic medicine. Consequently, there was faculty support for almost all the student proposals. The one area in which they didn't succeed was where the interests of some of the faculty diverged from those of the students: the proportion of time to be given various courses remained a function of the power of the different departments.

There were, though, a number of things the students did not ask for, like a curriculum more oriented towards social problems or revisions that would reduce the curriculum's tendency to socialize the students towards a particular set of values. They certainly did not ask for anything close to open-ended medical education available to all who sought it to whatever extent they desired. The final result was only some liberalization of the McGill course, carried out mostly by introducing some elective time and an opportunity to begin specializing before graduation (although, as I have indicated earlier in this chapter, this was by no means a fundamental change).

Another similar issue was popularly promoted during that time, centring on the introduction of a pass-fail system. Students were demanding change from a system that gave them relative rankings (upper, middle or lower-third of the class) to one that would merely indicate whether or not they had passed or failed: a change that had already been made by a majority of medical schools in North America. This was another chance for the students, almost all of whom backed the change, to show some solidarity. But here too the effort was only marginally successful. Student protest was tame, amounting largely to the signing of a petition. Most of the faculty lined up against the idea of change in the system, for a number of reasons. Many felt students would be at a disadvantage later on, especially when applying for internships, if there was not a record of their grades (ignoring the fact that almost all highly-regarded medical schools in the United States had already adopted pass-fail without stopping their own students from gaining positions, even at hospitals where competition was most fierce).* Others argued that a pass-fail system would not justly reward students who had done well (a concern that, on the whole, was not shared by the students). Some thought it might mean a lowering of McGill's standards.

A dean in charge of students' affairs, sympathetic to the idea of change, helped to win approval for a trial of pass-fail. But grading was not abandoned, merely withheld from view: marks were still recorded but not permitted to leave the Dean's office (although at the end of that year a computer printout was leaked from a university source outside the Dean's office; it included a calculation of percentage averages to one decimal point). In fact, grades remained as prominent as ever in the consciousness of the students and in their approach to their studies. Grades, however indirectly cited, continued to be a factor in the content of letters from the Dean in support of internship applications. In spite of this betrayal of what they had understood to be the intent of the pass-fail programme, not a whimper was heard from the students about it.*

During my time as student at McGill there were other issues that seemed to have more potential for organizing students and leading to some larger action. One of these was the "Lilly bag debate". It came up towards the end of first year, when our class learned we would be receiving a letter from the Eli Lilly company offering medical equipment: a stethoscope, a reflex hammer and a tuning fork, all neatly packaged in a doctor's bag. This equipment would be provided free to the students; all they had to do was return an enclosed business reply card to the company.

What was happening was fairly clear. Eli Lilly, one of the world's largest manufacturers of pharmaceutical products, was, like all major corporations, interested in maximizing its profits. To accomplish this it had to convince physicians and physicians-to-be to prescribe Lilly products frequently and in preference to those of other firms.

This was part, of course, of a more widespread phenomenon. Like other corporations, drug companies have resorted to massive campaigns of advertising and promotion in order to maintain their handsome annual return on investment.* Almost as much is now spent each year on drug promotion as on all medical education![26]

Pharmaceutical corporations have a higher advertising-to-sales ratio than does any other sector of the American economy.* All of this publicity and promotion is directed towards the people who can provide the market — the practising physicians, the physicians-in-training, and the medical students. Promotional efforts are slick and, often, unethical.[27]

While my class was confronting this issue, Eli Lilly was riding the crest of one of the most successful drug promotions in North American medical history, having propelled their so-called analgesic *Darvon* into the number one position on the Hit Parade of bestselling prescription drugs. They had not, however, been obliged to demonstrate the efficacy of this product and around 1970 articles began to appear indicating that *Darvon* was no more effective in killing pain than a placebo — a sugar pill — or, at best, two much less expensive aspirins.

But not many of us were yet reading medical journals and for most of us the gift of medical equipment from Lilly was to be our first contact with the marketing practices of pharmaceutical giants. Several members of the class thought that a principled position had to be taken in rejecting this attempted bribe — which the company insisted was nothing more than "good will" — if there was to be any hope of resisting the temptation of playing along with the drug companies at a later date by prescribing their products against the best interests of patients. These students suggested we send a collective letter to Eli Lilly, demanding that the offer not be made to the members of our class. A united front, they argued, would represent a significant victory.

Heated debate raged inside and outside every classroom. The students who favoured a boycott of the gifts continually buttonholed classmates, engaging them in discussion. Eventually, at a formal discussion held in class, the activists emphasized their well-known fear that the acceptance of the gifts would be the first step along the road to surrender to the drug companies in a war of attrition designed to win our allegiance on the prescription pad. Another group expressed the view that students could maintain independent judgement about pharmaceutical products even when they were receiving gifts from the manufacturers.

But the number of activists was relatively small and most of the class were apathetic (very few were downright hostile), rarely expressing much more than mild amusement at the fervour of the few. The indifference of this vast majority carried the day and there was no consensus achieved about boycotting the gifts. When the offers arrived, the students took their individual positions on the issue through the privacy of Her Majesty's mail. The next year, almost all were sporting Lilly equipment when they arrived on the hospital wards.

It is perhaps true that no decision our class might have taken on that occasion could have made much difference to what we would do later on as doctors: the Lilly bags were not the straw that broke the camel's back. The drug industry was not about to be prevented from spending nearly one billion dollars on marketing in North America each year. At best, a mass refusal of the equipment would have amounted to no more than symbolic opposition.

But acceptance of the gifts was symptomatic of two phenomena: the members of the class were being socialized into a particular world-view — if they did not already subscribe to it — and, more importantly, the socialization was occurring in a socio-economic order in which someone was offering a "gift" in the pursuit of profit. As for the debate itself, never again would so much emotion and electricity be discharged in the class; never again would a segment of the class be so aroused.

Another important issue that confronted my class was Medicare: the introduction of the Government-sponsored universal health insurance programme. The federal Government had offered to pay half the cost of any province's health insurance programme, providing it reached certain standards, and by the time the plan was introduced in the province of Quebec by a new Liberal Government in 1970, most of the other provinces had already adopted it. Quebec physicians were divided on the issue. General practitioners were happy with the financial settlement offered, so they endorsed the government programme. Not so the specialists, who were opposed to the principle as well as the particulars of Medicare. "Socialized medicine" was a bitter pill for the specialists to swallow; they were not about to be force-marched into the twentieth century.

It was not possible for the staff and students of the medical school to ignore the rapidly escalating crisis, for it was widely expected to result in a withdrawal of services by specialists. Almost all the teachers were members of the specialists' federation, which was being combative and menacing. In the Still and Quiet Air of Delightful Studies, the medical school faculty remained conspicuously silent.* And whatever their attitudes, most university specialists allowed the federation to speak for them. Those who supported Medicare kept quiet about it in public, although at some hospitals (the Royal Victoria in Montreal, for one) supporters of the legislation were very vocal and emotional in closed meetings with their colleagues.

Medicare was to be implemented in the autumn of 1970 and a strike of specialists was slated to coincide. While this crisis became a topic of conversation among the students, the tenor of discussion was mostly mild and academic. A clear majority of my classmates favoured the government programme, although many had some reservations. I found it surprising at the time that a substantial minority unequivocally opposed Medicare in principle. Some swallowed the specialists' line whole, defending the Profession, Freedom and Quality of Care.*

What was generally evident was that members of my class were less interested in the debate than were the practising members of the profession. Even when the strike seemed imminent there was no serious effort in the class to develop a collective position.*

Class members were, however, frequently exposed to the antagonism many of their teachers felt towards Medicare and this could not but help affect us. The practitioners had a good idea of what they thought the impact of Medicare would be, in fairly concrete terms: "I'm going to lose $10,000 a year" or "They aren't going to pay me as much as I deserve for each operation." As it happened, events subsequently demonstrated that they had overestimated the threat to their affluence.

What became apparent with this issue is the extent to which the students' perspectives were a function of how far they had progressed in their training. When Claude Castonguay, Quebec Minister of Health and centre of the storm, came at the height of the Medicare crisis to speak to the medical students, interns and residents, he attracted to the school's largest amphitheatre an overflow crowd of perhaps five hundred undergraduates and postgraduates. The audience was about evenly divided between supporters and opponents of Castonguay's legislation. He clearly had more support among the first and second year students in attendance than in the rest of the assembly. Most of the residents, interns and upper year students were antagonistic.* As students move closer to the practice of medicine their perspective becomes more and more that of the practitioners. (Some, of course, are faster "learners" than others, and develop the professional outlook much earlier.)

The reason for the difference in attitude of students in upper years who were hostile to Castonguay was only that they had been in medical school longer and had been more completely socialized into the values of the profession they were soon to join. In this sense, the initial perspective of students matters very little. Even students who have "progressive" values tend to be socialized no less relentlessly towards the professional outlook. It just might take them a little longer to get there.

During fourth year another minor crisis came up and it serves as one final example of aborted attempts at student activism. That year our class rotated in groups through the different clinical services in the university hospitals. In surgery — an eight-week stint — students were exposed to less teaching than we thought was our due. In fact, the rotation seemed to serve more as a chance for the hospitals to exploit students as cheap labour: our experience in the operating room consisted largely of pulling back on a patient's rib cage with a retractor while someone else did something just beyond our field of vision.

Because of this, many students felt that a surgery examination in fourth year was unnecessary. Besides, an oral examination the previous year had already probed our knowledge about theoretical (and some practical) aspects of the field. If a fourth year examination was to reflect what we learned that year, it should have tested our ability to draw blood, to insert intravenous tubing, to do admission physicals on pre-operative patients and to appear alert at seven in the morning: these were the ways in which we spent our time.

There was talk about the surgical oral but little action until two students flunked it. This meant an extra eight weeks of surgery for them, as well as a blemish on their records, and it frightened more than a few students. The next group of 23 students to rotate through surgery (which included me) wanted no part of it; we submitted a petition containing the signatures of all 23 students working the surgical wards of the two main teaching hospitals, indicating that we would not participate in an examination.

This raised some surgical eyebrows. A meeting was arranged between representatives of the students and the leading surgeons; the Associate Dean for students' affairs came along as arbitrator and chairman.

The surgeons began the meeting by taking the offensive, complaining that it was not reasonable "to change horses in midstream." They did indicate, though, that they might be willing to go along with some decrease in the value of the examination. Interpreting this as a show of weakness, we retorted that we were opposed to the idea of an examination, not just concerned with its value.

Surgeons are, in general, rather authoritarian people — even for physicians, and not easily cowed. But it appeared this time that the impressive solidarity of the students would lead to some sort of compromise. Then one student made the mistake of complaining about the surgery rotation in the mildest terms, observing that we were getting very little teaching. At this, one of the surgeons, a distinguished researcher with an international reputation, turned crimson and lost his temper.

"No one has ever talked to me that way!" he shouted. "How dare you! I don't have to listen to that kind of talk. I'm leaving." He flung a few more broadsides at the astonished student, then stormed from the room.

The rest of us looked on in stunned silence. The Associate Dean mumbled something about how nothing could be done about the examinations 'at this time', but added that the problem would be investigated further so that changes could be implemented for the benefit of future classes. We were enraged by the surgeon's incredible and immature behaviour.

Confounded, the representatives returned to the two hospitals with a proposal for a boycott. At first, everyone was prepared to go along, but one by one the militants backed down, until only a few were prepared to strike on examination day. This led finally to all resistance being abandoned and, ultimately, to unconditional surrender.

What caused this rapid erosion in principled fervour? One remark made by the surgeon during his outburst came very close to the answer. He said to the student criticising him: "You are a good student and I couldn't fail you, but I certainly wouldn't want you working on my service as an intern or resident."

This is exactly the problem. Even a little bit of trouble-making in medical school can jeopardize a career, and medical students are very career-conscious. Members of my class were acutely aware of the need to stay in the good graces of their professors in order to keep their career options open. This made any serious or extended protest beyond first year unlikely.

One McGill dental student put it most succinctly when admonishing his colleagues not to risk their careers for their principles. "Keep your nose clean and take lots of Valium," he said. And so they do. The surgeon's temper tantrum would not have been tolerated coming from a teacher in almost any other faculty, but it overwhelmed the future physicians. Self-interest was our motivation for protest; even greater self-interest was our justification for backing down.

What all these examples of attempts at student activism reveal is the difficulty of motivating and mobilizing medical students to move for change, no matter how minor. In the first place, the activism of my classmates was not directed towards changing either the social order or even its medical sector. The students were motivated in their actions, quite reasonably, by self-interest. Only very indirectly could their activism have benefited anyone else: if curriculum reform had enabled them to redirect towards societal problems the time previously wasted on destructive competition and unnecessary study. That was not their concern, however; they just wanted to make life more pleasant for themselves.

In fact, very few medical students have been deeply involved with social problems and even fewer have been prepared to do anything about them.* Reform in the medical school has rarely presented a serious challenge to prevailing medical ideology. Even when the "system" has been confronted, it has been most often a half-hearted effort, rapidly abandoned before the least resistance.

The truth is that the great majority of medical students stand to benefit economically, socially and culturally from the medical status quo. Few enter medical school with a perspective that is incompatible with such considerations, and those who do are given every incentive to abandon it.

Of course, the *subjective* justification is usually that medical studies leave insufficient time for broader concerns. Involvement with society's problems, with the priorities of medical education and medical practice, can be put aside and allowed to die gracefully while students concern themselves with more 'important' things like getting through the year and learning as much medicine as possible.

Whatever their world-views, students in medical school are made to feel the need to become competent practitioners in a relatively short time. With some justification, they give priority to this effort. Even those who maintain a progressive orientation frequently find themselves in the unsatisfactory position of supporting all the right causes and turning out for demonstrations and meetings, but not being seriously involved in efforts to develop or to implement radical analyses and strategies in medicine.

In the final result, the small number of people who survive their preclinical years with any politicization and social commitment are still more vulnerable to "rehabilitation" during the in-hospital training which takes place afterwards. Many do not even try to resist the gentle depoliticization (which is really politicization into a different ideology). For those who do make an effort to remain involved, the isolation from people of like mind and the lack of time to be politically active are obstacles that may prove impossible to overcome.

Call me Doctor: acquiring a professional consciousness

One of the most memorable moments in the career of medical students comes the day they are first addressed as "Doctor". For me, the Great Day came about midway through second year. Our class had just finished the bulk of our basic science courses (only pharmacology remained) and we were being given our first exposure to the hospital, a nine-week stint aptly named "Introduction to Clinical Science".

During this short course, we were expected to learn how to interview and examine a patient (an ambitious objective towards which most of us, hopefully, are still working). We were initially sequestered in groups where the basics of approaching the patient were explained to us. After a period of indoctrination, we were sent out into the "field", which consisted in my case of a small hospital affiliated with the medical school. I was assigned there along with three classmates to the tutelage of a young internist I will call Hassan.

Dr. Hassan's job was to take us around the wards of the hospital, teaching us the elucidation and interpretation of clinical signs and symptoms. He also had the task of assigning patients for us to "work up" — that is, for us to interrogate and examine. Finally, we would summarize our findings in a written report that included our impressions about diagnosis. Hassan was a good clinician and an excellent doctor. Watching him go through his motions was a pleasure; attempting to imitate him was fun. And it was not very far into that first day in his company that he began to address each of us as "Doctor".

The first time he addressed me that way was in the privacy of his office and I was mildly amused, if slightly disconcerted. When he referred to us all as "these young doctors" in the presence of a patient, I was terrified; I blushed (something I don't usually do) and I even thought momentarily of running from the room. "Surely the patient knows that isn't true," I thought. "He must be laughing to himself about this." One of the other students was visibly a bit off balance at that moment as well and a third admitted later to having been a little embarrassed. But we all managed to hold our ground.

This is all typical, it seems; students are usually first called Doctor around the time they begin their clinical training. Few students resist the designation, whatever reservations they may have about it. Those who do have objections oppose not the idea but the timing. Nevertheless, it is not infrequent for students to feel uncomfortable in the early stages when someone addresses them as Doctor. Later in their training, they will feel uncomfortable when someone does not.

That first day, the title certainly seemed inappropriate to our role and stage of training. After all, we were students who had only just emerged from our study of textbooks to look at patients for the very first time. We knew far less about recognizing disease than did the nurses, the orderlies or even many of the patients. We had been propelled into a status quite out of keeping with our competence, with an alacrity that at least some of us did not anticipate. There were good reasons for Hassan to call us doctors (which I shall discuss), but they were certainly not evident to me then.

But what soon did become evident was that the patients were willing to play along. They all knew we were neophytes (word quickly gets around a hospital ward about who's who), but they accorded us the deference due to members of the medical profession and regularly took the trouble to address each of us as Doctor, taking their cue from Hassan.

The patients thus fell into the trap of mystifying themselves about us. That is, they placed us in a category apart — a category of individuals who are generally given credit for more knowledge and ability than they possess, and to whom many people surrender power over important aspects of their lives.

Being *called* Doctor is only part of *being* a doctor, however, and the acquisition of a professional identity is as important in student development as the acquisition of a title. Not all students don their doctor identity at the same time. Some have it from the first day they set foot in medical school; others develop it soon thereafter. A few never really accept the identity (even if they play the part) and are looked upon as maladjusted or insecure.

It is one thing to feel secure in an abstract medical identity when sitting in a library or lecture theatre. It is something else, however, to deal confidently and 'professionally' with patients and health workers under the actual title of Doctor. Students can experience new and profound trauma at this stage, because they do not approach patients as apprentices but as people who have already begun to assume a professional identity.

For the better part of two years, physicians-to-be have spent most or all of their time in the company of medical students. Even their social life has been medically-oriented.* On and on it goes: the medical classroom, the medical library, the medical party, the medical date... Even conversations and encounters with non-medical people are co-opted, since so many dearly want to pluck some medical knowledge — a rare commodity in lay society — from the brain of some available pluckee.

Those who enter the hospitals in second year to learn how to examine patients are more than medical students. They are part of a medical sub-culture. They are looked upon by family, friends and classmates as some approximation of a physician (after all, it is just a matter of time). Not only have they begun to acquiesce in their professional identity; they have become dependent upon it for diminishing their anxieties, for structuring their relationships and so on. Thus they approach patients with some conception of themselves as Doctor even though their clinical judgement is probably no better than that, say, of their mothers, who usually have at least some experience in caring for the sick.

What is perhaps most frightening for students during this early exposure to clinical medicine is the possibility that they will not convey the impression of possessing at least some of the physician's competence. Were it not for their need to appear competent and professional to their patients, students would not be terrified about forgetting to review the musculoskeletal system when interviewing a patient, or about admitting that they cannot see the blood vessels when examining a patient's eye with an ophthalmoscope: a person has to learn some time.

The desire to impress others derives from a need to convince themselves of the validity and immutability of their identities as physicians. So important has this become that the possibility that they will fail to live up to their own expectations is frightening indeed. When the title of Doctor is thrown in, the stakes become that much higher.

The decision about when the title should be conferred is not the the students' to make, except to the extent that they may encourage or facilitate it. It is the hospital physicians, the teachers, who decide when to address their disciples as physicians.

Why do these others do it? Is it part of some diabolical conspiracy on the part of the medical school to condition the students to the role they will subsequently play as the aristocrats of the health care system? Even though one result of the treatment students receive from superiors is that their perspective becomes even more coloured by the profession's outlook, there is no organized or even conscious effort to make them think and act like Doctors. On the contrary, the approach taken seems natural and logical to the physician-teachers for a number of reasons.

Often physicians will address their students as Doctor in the belief that this will make it easier for them to function in the context of the hospital. It makes life simpler for the physician-teachers as well, particularly if they are not familiar with the names of all the students who are accompanying them on a particular day. Another reason the designation seems appropriate is that many physicians feel patients should believe that the person who is examining them is, in fact, a physician, or something more than just a student with a beginner's rudimentary knowledge of medical problems.* For other hospital workers, it is alleged, it simplifies the work situation if they are able to deal with everyone wearing a white coat and sporting a stethoscope as Doctor. This is true, but it also accomplishes the rigid structuring of work relationships.

Some students in my class reported that in some of their early experiences on the wards they were called Doctor in a most sarcastic and condescending way by physicians who were thus expressing intolerance for their juniors' ignorance. Physicians patronize their students in another way when they bestow the coveted title: it magnifies their self-importance to be able to do so. Besides bolstering the teacher's ego, this act of generosity presumably makes students feel somehow indebted to their "benefactor".

Of course, the students do not always experience this largesse in the way teachers expect them to. I don't remember feeling any indebtedness, only astonishment and terror, when Hassan first addressed me as Doctor. He did, however, leave a considerable impression on myself and the others by so doing. Hassan was an Iranian whose accent seemed specifically tailored to linger over such words as 'Doctor'. One of my most vivid recollections of second year is of him standing there saying "Duawk-tair Roberts, Duawk-tair Smith, Duawk-tair Schwartz, Duawk-tair Shapiro."

Whatever our initial reaction to this precipitous introduction to our professional roles, the long-term implications were quite acceptable to most of us. Henceforth, all our interactions in the hospital would be as physicians. Our titles would explicitly legitimize what our behaviour would implicitly dictate. By mediating our relationships with nurses, patients, and others through our newly acquired identities, all our relationships would thereby be structured through the hospital hierarchy. Making interactions predictable in this way would be a happy outcome for many of us, by ultimately reducing the anxiety we felt in the hospital.

It is ironic that the professional role (and its accompanying title) which can provoke so much anxiety at first, actually diminishes it in the end. The initial problem is really only one of adjustment, however, and once students have made that adjustment, things flow very smoothly. The world becomes a far less complicated place for those who can say "Call me Doctor". Of course, they pay a price for this identity: the likelihood of ever exploring alternative, spontaneous, creative modes of relating to patients and others is considerably diminished. Nevertheless, few consider this to be much of a drawback, as can be understood in the context of that popular approach to human relationships propounded in the mass-marketed writings of Norman Vincent Peale:

1. Formulate and stamp indelibly on your mind a mental picture of yourself as succeeding. Hold this picture tenaciously. Never permit it to fade. Your mind will seek to develop this picture. Never think of yourself as failing; never doubt the reality of the mental image. That is most dangerous, for the mind always tries to complete what it pictures. So always picture 'success' no matter how badly things seem to be going at the moment.
2. Whenever a negative thought of your personal powers comes to mind, deliberately voice a thought to cancel it out.[28]

Dr. Peale's strategy for coping is not unlike that used by the medical student. The corollaries are: do not examine your relationships with others in a critical way; do not consider the implications of your activity and the alternatives to it; do not consider the extent to which your anxieties and aspirations are functions of an environment that is not unchangeable; instead, develop a very positive *image* of yourself (however unrealistic or unhealthy it may be) that will permit you to repress anxieties rather than seek their causes and their solutions. This is a prescription for accepting the values of society, and for acquiescing in socialization into a role that is a function of those values.

Significantly, this structuring is often more beneficial to doctors than to those they relate to, for it allows them to assume a position of dominance. But the benefit is only superficial. While doctors may derive reassurance and comfort from their professional identity when confronting the strangers they call patients in the big, intimidating hospital, they also accept the limited perspective inherent in their identity. (The outlook of nurses undergoes similar regimentation in nursing school.)[29] They surrender the potential for seriously and critically examining the medical environment and their role within it.

Unable to understand the implications of the hospital experience for others (however 'positive' it may be for themselves), they forgo the possibility of developing alternatives. Their mechanism of adaptation stands opposed to any development of more humane social and personal relations. Even those students who are aware of this problem are nonplussed by it. Indeed, theirs is a rather common mechanism for coping in modern society. As R.D. Laing observes:

Human beings seem to have an almost unlimited capacity to deceive themselves and to deceive themselves into taking their own lies for truth. By such mystification, we achieve and sustain our adjustment, adaptation, socialization.[30]

Student physicians, by following a well-trodden road through difficult terrain, come to believe that it is the only road. Their professional identity may comfort them at times, and it may also be exactly what some patients and others are looking for in them but, more than anything else it accomplishes, it dictates the terms of their subsequent work activity.

My classmates and I did not remain anxious or uncomfortable in our new identities for very long. Within a few weeks, we felt no anxiety at being addressed as 'Duawk-tair' in front of a patient. By the time my course with Hassan had ended, I had learned to expect most people in the hospital to call me Doctor and even to treat me as such on occasion.

At first, only a few students had the nerve to introduce themselves to the patients as Doctor. Most of us were either non-committal (using unqualified surnames) or honest ("My name is . . . I am a second year medical student. Do you mind if I examine you?")

In third year, however, few students would approach patients without identifying themselves as Doctor. That year was spent almost entirely in the hospitals as we rotated through surgery, psychiatry and internal medicine. We met resident physicians, ate in the hospital cafeteria, drank coffee in the interns' and residents' lounge. At this point it was possible to begin to think concretely of being and becoming physicians.

By fourth year, there was further progress into the physician identity. Fourth-year students expected to be introduced as Doctor at all times, and might well become upset if not treated accordingly. Rare was the person who would not have considered it a major insult to be introduced to a patient as "student".*

During fourth year we functioned more or less as interns. Calling us Doctor was the accepted practice for the resident staff, and not only to make us happy. It was thought inappropriate that patients be made aware of the fact that the person in white who came to see and examine them each day (their 'primary care physician') was in reality, only a student!

Thus did our expectations change dramatically as we progressed through medical school. The original reticence in accepting the professional mantle was more a matter of stagefright than of conviction.* Most members of the class had learned well by fourth year how to play the part fearlessly and with many of its subtleties: paternalism, aloofness, omnipotence. Anxieties were not overcome or resolved, but repressed through the consolidation of a professional identity that provided a large measure of protection from self-doubt. The escape of student physicians from anxiety is only as good as their hiding place. Were their professional disguise stripped away, their original dilemma would confront them once again.

But just as the escape from anxiety is in no way a cure, the event which crystallized that anxiety was not really the cause. The need of medical students for identification as physicians is not at all inappropriate in a society in which many people are desperately seeking just such an identity. The desire to structure one's relations with others in a way that is favourable to oneself is not aberrant behaviour, although it is far from liberating.

In a society that denies fulfillment in so many important ways, people feel compelled to elevate themselves in their own esteem at all costs. Medical students can accomplish this by capitalizing upon an opportunity to assume an identity that places them in a position of superiority over others. Driven by unhealthy and oppressive relationships in the medical school and the medical hierarchy, egged on by the expectations of parents and friends and by needs derived from outside the medical context, students allow this need for self-esteem to be transmuted into a lust for power — the power of the physician. As Erich Fromm suggests, this is not a healthy sign:

[T]he lust for power is not rooted in strength but in weakness. It is an expression of the inability of the individual self to stand alone and live. It is the desperate attempt to gain secondary strength where genuine strength is lacking.[31]

The desire to assume the physician identity, then, derives from weakness, fragility and insecurity. That they do seek this power over others is not a disease particular to medical students; according to Fromm such strivings, when prevalent in society, are not a sign of disease in the individual. What makes the students' situation different from that of many others is that their feelings of weakness and inadequacy are so greatly intensified by the context in which they work and study. Furthermore, they are given a channel of escape, through a 'legitimate' exercise of power over others, to which few in society have access (exceptions including police, prison guards, teachers). They do not have to exercise this power, of course, but the temptations are strong.

Undoubtedly, the idealism that some students hold is diminished by their experiences in medical training. Hard work, competition and the other factors contribute to the socialization of the physician into the values of the profession. But it should be added that medical school cannot bear the entire blame. In a society that encourages its members to accumulate as much as possible, even at the expense of others, and in which there is little importance placed on humane interpersonal relations, many forces help to socialize the physician besides what happens within the medical school and the hospital. The alienation of the physician cannot be understood as resulting solely from an educational experience, when all relations within society are alienated.

Notes

page 27: In fact, even one year in medical school was enough to make me a *Medical Student,* and not merely someone who had been studying medicine for a year. My father marked my progress at the end of the year by calling me "one-quarter of a doctor". In terms of my professional consciousness, at least, this was an underestimate. Although he did not live to see me graduate, my father saw more of the finished product than he probably realized.

page 30a: The medical school does much to foster these tendencies. A calendar of classes given to us during first year described a combined course in microbiology, pathology and epidemiology to be given during the forthcoming year. The book listed the time, location and subject matter of every lecture that would be given. One afternoon each week was not scheduled for classes or laboratories; it was listed as "Dean's Free Time". The designation was apt, for this "free time" certainly provided no respite from our involvement in matters medical.

30b: I remember one encounter during first year, with a fourth-year meds student whom I had known for some time outside medicine. "How are things going on lower campus?" he asked. (The medical school and the hospitals are on higher ground than the undergraduate buildings at McGill.) "Fine," I replied. "Now you know," he continued, "why it is that we call it 'lower campus'."

page 31: Medical teachers are rarely willing to tell students when they are *not* responsible for something. (See H.S. Becker, B. Geer, E.C. Hughes, A.L. Strauss: *Boys in White* [Chicago: University of Chicago Press, 1961] pp89-90.)

page 32: In my class there were students who did not work irrationally hard. They were not necessarily more admirable than those who did — some of them were just lazy. In any event, compulsive, excessive studying was widely prevalent, and it, more than anything else, typified the class's orientation.

page 37a: This statistic was cited to me by a despondent physiology professor who believed, along with many others, that anatomy was being over-taught. For reasons I shall explore, he was unable to do anything about this imbalance.

37b: Many did not even do that much, because time spent at epidemiology was regarded as time away from pathology and microbiology, which were examined at the same time.

page 38: This was not as much of a problem in Europe, where the use of cadavers was accepted by the public much earlier.

page 39: It may well be that some day anatomy will become a minor course at McGill. It may even be undertaught, although that is hard to imagine. But if this kind of change does occur, it will be because the power and influence of the anatomy department have diminished in the councils of the medical faculty.

page 42: Similar dynamics exist in the law school classroom, as was well illustrated by the film *Paper Chase*. The film's protagonist describes a functional breakdown of his class that applies not less to my medical class. A small number of students actively participate. Others are reluctant to participate but do respond when called upon. Still others have given up altogether on any kind of involvement in the law school classroom. In the law school, just as in medical school, a hierarchy of knowledge exists; all the students know, or think they know, just where they stand in that hierarchy.

page 43: This reminds me of Koko in *The Mikado*, giving his fiancee to another to save his own neck:

Now I adore that girl with passion tender and could not yield her with a ready will, or her allot, if I did not adore myself with passion tenderer still!

page 44: This game of one-upmanship is also played by interns and residents, who are likewise graded by others each step of the way. An intern at a San Francisco hospital where I worked as a student was said by his colleagues to have bribed the hospital mailman to hold back for a few days everyone else's copy of *The New England Journal of Medicine* — so he could impress others by quoting the latest article before anyone else had a chance to read it.

page 45: In *Boys in White*, the authors show that students acquire this attitude in the very first months of medical school. (See H.S. Becker, B. Geer, E.C. Hughes, A.L. Strauss, *Boys in White* [Chicago: University of Chicago Press, 1961], pp92-184.)

page 46: The obsession with certification and with the passing of examinations does not end with graduation from medical school. At UCLA Hospital in Los Angeles, where it is an unusual year when *anyone* fails the internal medicine specialty certification examination, I heard colleagues talk anxiously about their prospects on that examination from the first day I set foot in the hospital until the day we received the test results. Everyone, including some very bright physicians, expressed fear of failing from time to time. Nor did any of us receive with anything like equanimity the predictable letter of congratulations from the American Board of Internal Medicine!

page 47a: Some of my classmates used to talk about what to do with an elective block that was two years away. They were really quite crafty: a student who did three or four electives in internal medicine subspecialties at a particular hospital was well on the way to an appointment there as an intern.

47b: Electives narrow the focus of students, quite the opposite of what some hoped would be accomplished. In this respect, McGill is to be congratulated for being one of the few schools to stop playing the game quite so self-righteously. McGill has reduced "elective" time and has designated as electives such essentials as courses in alcoholism, human sexuality and the dying patient, courses almost all the students take. But McGill also has introduced "selectives", which are early opportunities to specialize and to focus interest; that is, what electives have effectively been used for all along.

page 50: Besides the MCHR, a research and documentation group in New York, the Health Policy Advisory Committee (Health/PAC), has churned out reams of cogent criticism of the American health system. It opened a second office in San Francisco that was later closed because of political disagreements.

page 53a: One factor motivating this concern for their students may have been a fear felt by some academics that they would not be able to continue boosting their egos by landing prestigious internships for their 'boys'.

53b: With the waning of student activism, medical schools are starting to drop their pass-fail systems. This tendency has recently been blessed by the medical education establishment. (See D.D. Federman, "Will pass/fail pass?", *New England Journal of Medicine* 299 [1978]: 43-44.)

53c: At a rate of profit on the order of 20 per cent per year, the American pharmaceutical industry is one of the best performers in the economy, doing twice as well as manufacturers as a whole. (See N. Doherty, "Excess profits in the drug industry and their effect on consumer expenditures", *Inquiry* 10 [September 1973]: 19-30.)

page 54: At 15.4 per cent, it ranks even ahead of the soaps and detergents industry, whose unrelenting media barrages are familiar to all. (See M.J. Murray, "The Pharmaceutical Industry: a study in corporate power", *International Journal of Health Services* 4, no.4 [1974]: 625-640.)

page 55: "In the Still and Quiet Air of Delightful Studies" is from an inscription on the wall of McGill's Redpath Library.

page 56a: This was not out of line with attitudes that medical students have generally held to health services reform. When Medicare for the aged was introduced in the United States, many medical students opposed it, usually without detailed knowledge of the legislation.

56b: Becker and his colleagues hypothesize that the attitude of students to medical practice is a synthesis of the perspectives of the public and of the profession. (See H.S. Becker, et.al., *op.cit.* pp89-91.) In the case of my class, it would seem that the perspective of the profession significantly influenced the students. In fact, no synthesis was possible. The professional and the public interests stood clearly opposed, with the students caught somewhere in the middle.

56c: Confirming this, the organization representing interns and residents in the province declared itself opposed to Medicare. (See M. Taylor, "Quebec Medicare policy formation in conflict and crisis", *Canadian Public Administration* 15, no.2 [1972]: 211-250.)

page 59: Fitzhugh Mullan has written a moving memoir of the radical health movement in the 1960s, in which he played a major role both as a medical student and resident physician. While granting that he and his colleagues failed to achieve radical change, even in terms of their limited objectives of the day (for the most part, to orient medicine more towards the poor urban communities), Mullan does see changes in the last ten years that he regards as significant. He believes that medical schools have become more progressive and that this is being reflected in the profession; that young physicians "look and act" differently from older colleagues; that the medical profession is less of a monolith in lifestyle and outlook than he supposes it at one time to have been; that the profession has "room for people who want to work in ghettos and on reservations, who like to smoke dope and live collectively, who prefer salaries to fee-for-service"; and that fee-for-service private practice is no longer the standard for American medicine. He concludes that "the middle-aged, conservative, free-enterprise, anti-labour hegemony in the profession no longer exists". Some of Mullan's "changes" never took place; I leave it to the reader to judge the extent to which those that did can be considered truly significant and progressive. (See Fitzhugh Mullan, *White Coat, Clenched Fist: The Political Education of an American Physician* [New York: Macmillian, 1976], pp215-222.)

page 61: The parties they attend as a respite from studying, which are organized by members of their class, regularly attract hordes of nursing and other paramedical students.

page 62: In the later years of medical school, students do more than examine patients, they also care for them. A large proportion of patients in university hospitals are under the care of students. I discuss this problem in greater detail in chapter five.

page 65a: Female students were, if anything, more anxious to assume the mantle of physician and, thereby, to clarify in the minds of patients, other health workers and themselves that they were a class apart from the nurses.

65b: Huntington has documented this transition in student attitude at three American medical schools. She found that 30 per cent of the students thought of themselves "primarily as doctors" as early as first year; by graduation day, this figure had reached 83 per cent. (See M.J. Huntington, "The development of a professional self-image", in R.K. Merton, G.G. Reader, P.L. Kendall, *The Student Physician: Introductory Studies in the Sociology of Medical Education* [Cambridge: Mass.: Harvard University Press, 1957], pp179-187.)

3

On Receiving Knowledge

The attitudes of medical students towards the learning process evolve almost predictably as their education proceeds. Conned at first into believing they must know everything there is to know, eventually they come to the realization that what they really have to learn is only what is asked about in examinations.

H.C. Becker and the other authors of the book *Boys in White* studied this phenomenon as it applied to medical students at the University of Kansas in the late fifties.[1] The four authors found that while many students were quite idealistic when arriving at the school, intending to learn as much as possible in preparation for medical practice, they soon began to show concern about their inability to "keep up" with the work. Within a couple of months most of the students had abandoned their efforts to learn as much as possible. While still suffering from that "compulsion to overwork" discussed in the previous chapters, they cynically oriented their study activity solely towards examinations.

Because of this examination orientation, an "underground" developed, much to the consternation of the faculty. The students copied assignments and evolved shortcuts to studying and preparing for examinations. This allowed them to amass in readily regurgitable form, the factual knowledge they would need in the examination room:

[T]eaching methods that do not approach the concrete finality of a textbook seem wasteful to the students. They think of medicine as a tremendous body of facts that they must learn. Their efforts are so directed towards entering the examination room knowing these facts, that they do many things along the way that the faculty does not like.[2]

Stampeded by the anxiety that examinations provoke, medical

students — in my class no less than in the Kansas group — rapidly abandon whatever perspective they bring with them to the school and collectively accept the struggle to survive.

Tools for learning

The strategies for survival employed by medical students do not vary greatly from place to place or from year to year. An important part of the process is the storing of data in readily retrievable form, and a favourite technique for doing this is the **mnemonic**. For instance:

Lovely French Tart Sitting Naked in Anticipation. The first letters of each word in this phrase represent (in ascending order) the seven major branches of the external carotid artery.

Ten Zebras Bit My Cock Off. The first letters represent the branches of the facial nerve.

Thick-Thighed Ladies Live In Place Ville-Marie. The eight essential amino acids.

Fuck Right Off. The orifices through which the three branches of the trigeminal nerve emerge from the skull.

An obvious feature of these mnemonics is their sexual (and sexist) orientation. Some commentators have referred to this use of 'dirty' phrases as an intellectualization of the students' anxieties about confronting death, particularly in the form of the cadaver. This may be part of the truth, but the mnemonics also indicate something about attitudes to male-female relationships.

Student use of devices like mnemonics also offers considerable insight into attitudes to learning. The irrelevance of first year subjects, for instance, is no great secret in medical school. Almost all first year students have some friends or acquaintances in the upper years or come into contact with upperclassmen as the year progresses; from these people come assurances that the courses in anatomy, histology and biochemistry are of minimal importance in subsequent training. As a result, the students want to put in the minimal amount of time necessary for learning what they need to know.

But devices like mnemonics should be recognized for what they are: shortcuts to prepration for examinations, not shortcuts to knowledge. They do not increase comprehension: learning in this way the essential amino acids has *no* utility beyond their regurgitation in an exam. (Students who understand the metabolism of the amino acids, on the other hand, do not need mnemonics to remind them which ones are essential.) I have to admit that in writing this chapter, I can recall the sexist ditties above far better than I do the quanta of medical "knowledge" they were intended to represent.

Unfortunately, comprehension is not a serious objective of most studying in medical school. Students do not have to learn deductively and retain information indefinitely; all they have to do is cram the material in and spew it forth on the fateful day. When fulfilling the examiner's demands is all that students are concerned with, it is only appropriate that they learn by rote.

The mnemonic was not the only technique we had for efficiently arraying in our minds facts that could be later plucked out during examinations. When I recently checked my *Grant's Atlas of Anatomy* to look up the branches of the external carotid artery mentioned above, I found a few sheets of paper that were extremely valuable to me in first year. On these pages were summarized all the questions that had been asked on anatomy practical examinations in the few years prior to my encounter with the course.

I was a latecomer to this valuable tool in the crammer's bag of tricks. Some of my classmates made a science of it and had extensive files of such questions, going back ten years or even more. The University of Kansas students of *Boys in White* were even more systematic. Their three medical fraternities had extensive files of previous examinations.[3] Similarly, at medical schools where the United States National Board examinations count towards grades, 'pre-test' books containing many hundreds of examination-type questions sell very well.

It may seem even more crass and pragmatic for the students to study examination papers than to use memory aids such as mnemonics, but it is really just an extension of the same process. From the format of the exams as well as from the recent track record of specific questions, it is possible to anticipate many of the questions that will be asked. Some appear every year; others every two or three years. You could safely ignore a substantial section of course content if that section did not fit into the examination format. On the other hand, a less important area would be closely studied if it were known to be a favourite of the examiner. My class knew, for example, that on the anatomy practical examination we would almost certainly be asked to identify the conjoined tendon. Or, on the histology exam there was usually one major essay question each year, dealing with the cellular structure of the liver or the kidney. All of this means that, while medical school teachers might officially discourage students from being too examination-oriented, professional emphasis on the importance of doing well on tests makes it almost certain that examinations will dominate the lives of the students.

Of course, the pragmatic approach to examinations is neither surprising nor unusual. Anyone who is forced to study a certain subject under a system based on external compulsion might be expected to do the same. And, at every turn, study activity fails to fulfill students, even in the limited ways they hope. The more they concern themselves with strategies, the more anxious they get and the further removed from their conception of what they originally set out to learn (All There Is To Know, Everything That Will Be Useful, or whatever). The study activity becomes only a very indirect means to an end: it permits students to acquire the credits needed in order to graduate from medical school, but it has relatively little to do with developing the skills necessary for the practice of medicine. Their work amounts to little more than surmounting a series of obstacles; in the process they become less sensitive to people and problems external to this work setting, and they even begin to accept the legitimacy of the games they are playing and the limitations of that experience. In important ways, their examination-centred work compromises and diminishes their sense of their own possibilities, along with their ability to realize them.

The upshot is that medical students do not engage in study for its own sake — to learn— but because they believe study is necessary in order to obtain what they want. This situation falls close to the one described by Karl Marx in his discussion of the relationship of workers to the product of their labour:

[T]he worker is related to the product of his labour as to an alien object. For it is clear that the more the worker spends himself. . . the poorer he himself — his inner world — becomes, the less belongs to him as his own . . . . The worker puts his life into the object; but now his life no longer belongs to him but to the object. Hence, the greater this activity, the greater is the worker's lack of objects.

His labour is therefore not voluntary but coerced; it is forced labour. It is not the satisfaction of a need; it is merely a means to satisfy a need external to it.[4]

This is what Marx calls the alienation of the worker.* And, while workers cannot attempt to realize their potential and express their individuality through work on an assembly line, medical students too deny their individual creativity and spontaneity in the working conditions they have accepted. They follow certain dictates and, in effect, contract to memorize a certain number of facts in exchange for the seal of progress. Their work is not a spontaneous effort to fulfill themselves; it is also not primarily directed towards the acquisition of an education; it is the fulfilment of a requirement established for them by others.

Learning on the ward

When, finally, medical students escape from classrooms and arrive on the wards of hospitals, they are still not freed from the need to concentrate on gathering data. And the data are still being compiled, largely so they can be displayed to advantage in settings only slightly different from examinations.

The Professor, who can be distinguished by the length of his white coat, is touring the ward in the company of a few students. They are discussing a case of splenomegaly (enlargement of the spleen).

"Why do you think this man has splenomegaly, Jones?" he asks one of the students.

"Well, the chances are it is related to his liver cirrhosis, which has caused portal hypertension," Jones replies.

"What other causes of splenomegaly are you familiar with, Jones?"

"Uh, well, there's infectious mononucleosis, hepatitis, lymphoma, leukemias, some anemias. Those are the important ones."

"What else?"

"Uh . . . "

"Smith, you tell Jones the differential diagnosis of splenomegaly," snaps the Professor.

"There's lymphangioma, hemangioma, post-traumatic enlargement, portal or splenic vein thrombosis, cirrhosis, thrombocytopenic purpura, hemolytic anemia, iron deficiency anemia, Cooley's anemia, pernicious anemia, hyperthyroidism, Gaucher's Disease, Niemann-Pick Disease, amyloidosis, SLE, Still's Disease, Felty's Syndrome, serum sickness, sarcoidosis . . ."

"Very good. You certainly seem to know your work. Jones, you ought to familiarize yourself with this differential diagnosis."

"What about this case?" asks another student.

"Oh," says the Professor, "it's obviously cirrhosis of the liver."

Just as preclinical students must be able to regurgitate prescribed facts on an examination, so must clinical trainees be ready and able to cough up differential diagnoses on demand. It matters not how relevant the various diagnoses are to the case at hand; it is the performance that counts.

In defence of the maligned Jones, it must be said that it is possible to provide patients with exemplary care without being able to rattle off the names of a dozen relatively rare conditions. Jones, in fact, names the important and relevant ones. If he had attempted to deduce other possibilities from the theory he knew, he could have expanded his list. Beyond that, he could have looked up the differential diagnosis of splenomegaly in any of several textbooks that contain comprehensive listings. Certainly, if the focus of his exchange with the professor was only to learn medicine and to provide the patient with good care, this approach would suffice. But students like Jones are playing a highly competitive game and, if they want to get good interning positions, they have to take the game as seriously as their classmates and work at rehearsing their act.

The Professor (a staff or attending physician) is making rounds on the ward with the house officers. An intern is presenting a case.

"Mrs. Rale is a sixty-four-year old woman with a history of coronary artery disease and two myocardial infarctions [heart attacks]. *She was delivered to the emergency room last night with acute pulmonary oedema. We gave her 80 milligrams of furosemide intravenously and she responded well. We have started her on digitalis. There was an interesting article in* The New England Journal of Medicine *on August 14, 1975 in which Friedman and his colleagues reported on two cases of unilateral pulmonary oedema after renal transplantation."*

The Professor's face lights up. "Very interesting," he says. "Why don't you put a copy of the article in the chart? It sounds like we should all read it. Next case."

By citing 'the literature', this house officer polishes off a virtuoso performance and scores even more points with the professor evaluating him. One member of my class did astonishingly well by citing the same article on pancreatitis to several of his teachers.

Predictably, the mnemonic also finds its way into these bedside spectacles. One student I know used one to memorize 37 causes of splenomegaly, thereby propelling himself towards the internship of his choice.

Rarely in physician training does anyone pay much attention to the ability to relate to patients, or even to the ability to examine them properly. But if students are unable to give an 'adequate' differential diagnosis, or quote an 'interesting' article, then watch out. In my third year, the class was expected to demonstrate our clinical prowess by reciting differential diagnoses. In fourth year this was not enough; we had to be able to quote the literature as well.

One resident complained to me that whenever he was called in to help with the evaluation of medical students, all the professors wanted to know was: "Does the student read the literature?" A student's ability to do work on the ward did not interest them.

The effects of this alienated activity on students are not transitory. Many continue to behave in the same way in their later careers. The regard that academic physicians hold for their colleagues has little to do with ability to teach or care for patients, but more for their worth as performers.

One resident I worked with used to express disapproval of colleagues by saying, "He hasn't got facts." This was his ultimate insult. Such was his perception — and that of many others — of what the physician should be all about. And students who emphasize the amassing of facts become physicians oriented towards the collection of data. They are trained to observe and to describe. They are more concerned with determining the cause of illness than its cure.

The person with such a perspective will be more interested in disease than in health, more interested in diagnosis than in therapy. Physicians are so conditioned to an empahsis on facts that they are most comfortable when they can approach their work in this way. It is easy to imagine from this how patients can lose their human identity in the medical setting and come to be seen as a collection of data to be analysed. If the data are not interesting to the physician, the physician will not show much interest in the patient.

Learning the "exceptional" case

The majority of people who go to see a physician in our society do so because of an emotional problem or a minor complaint, such as an upper respiratory tract infection. The medical school curriculum does not emphasize the treatment of these disorders (and consequently many physicians end up mistreating them). Nor does it emphasize other relatively common and important problems, such as hypertension and alcoholism. The focus of the curriculum is that which delights the medical school teacher (and the students as well): the exceptional problem.

I am sure that my class received more instruction on disease entities such as systemic lupus erythematosis, polyarteritis nodosa, and sarcoidosis than we did on heart attacks. Our professors loved to talk about wayout diseases, and everyone in the class knew what lupus did to the kidney long before Marcus Welby told the American public about it. The pathological effects of these diseases on body structures and processes were elegantly described to us. We also learned the pathological implications of more common disorders but, since there was a limited amount to be said and these disorders were relatively easy to diagnose, they were not given emphasis in proportion to their importance. The teaching staff apparently did not feel it was important to drill students repeatedly on the essentials of these problems. That would have been boring for all concerned.

Much of the work of physicians is repetitious and straightforward. Because of this physicians enjoy investigating patients with unusual problems: those problems stimulate and challenge the intellect, they are less routine, and they make the work more bearable. Thus patients with high blood pressure are often ignored, even though the disease is potentially fatal,[5] while patients with a bizarre symptom complex will receive the "super-workup" in the hope of uncovering a rare and "interesting" disease. The fact that many of the unusual conditions are less susceptible to therapy does not deter the physicians. Even when a person with hypertension does attract their interest, it is as a diagnostic problem — the search for an occasional case with a rare cause — rather than a therapeutic one; this in spite of the fact that most studies indicate hypertension can be effectively treated without respect to the cause.*

The ultimate expression of the physician's orientation to the "exceptional" data and diagnosis is found in the pages of *The New England Journal of Medicine*. Every week, the NEJM publishes a "clinical-pathological conference", where a case history is presented with an expert in the field discussing the differential diagnosis and attempting to predict the "anatomical findings" at autopsy or operation (where the patients involved invariably end up). The case is almost always an "interesting" one, meaning that it involves a rare disease or that the diagnosis is otherwise unexpected. The discussant, if any good at all, will put on a dazzling performance, gliding gracefully through dozens of possible diagnoses, and finally disclosing how it was deduced that the patient — who was going to die in any event — had one tumor rather than another.

Medical student and practitioner alike love these "exercises" because it feeds them what they think are the significant aspects of medicine. These aspects have not much to do with what physicians confront in their offices every day, but they do satisfy the need for diversity and intellectual stimulation so often lacking in the job.

Learning: the professional mystique

Physicians imagine themselves scientists of sorts, and it is the scientific inquiry in their work that most often captures their imaginations. There has long been a tendency in medical practice for physicians to play the part of observer and recorder at least as much as healer. This approach dates from classical antiquity and was systematized when Abraham Flexner and his report established the "scientific basis" of medical education. It is now the mainstay of medical practice in North America. Unfortunately, the approach is only beneficial to the rare patient with a rare condition. People who go to their doctors with "garden variety" complaints may be unaware that they are not living up to the physicians' expectations.

If the learning involved in becoming a physician were oriented primarily towards benefitting the patient, the emphasis on diagnosis as well as most of the facts the students assimilate in their first two years could be discarded. Then, however, physicians would have difficulty maintaining their status as professionals holding valuable and exclusive knowledge sought by others.

Thus in medical education there is some method in the madness of mnemonics, examinations, differential diagnoses and the rest. While most of the knowledge gained is of only marginal relevance to the actual practice of medicine (one member of my class came back from an elective period with some general practitioners in Newfoundland convinced that *anyone* could learn in a month everything necessary to do the work of a GP), physicians who have processed tens of thousands of facts through their brains are able to convey the impression of knowing a great deal about something important. This is their professional mystique: the physician as omnipotent and omniscient.

Physicians rarely admit to ignorance because their image of infinite ability to process patient data would be tarnished by such a confession of failure. Students learn this early. One Boston-area student told me about an encounter he had with a professor, who asked him a question about some disease.

"I don't know", he told the professor.

"You don't know! That is not a Harvard medical student answer," snorted the physician-teacher.

The education of physicians is intended to provide them with both medical skills and medical knowledge, and it manages to confuse the two. The most important thing to be learned about a large spleen is how and when one should look for it in the course of examining a patient, and how it is to be recognized as enlarged — something many physicians cannot do properly. Beyond this, the investigation of a patient with splenomegaly is a matter of following a recipe in a textbook. While a certain amount of understanding of the biochemical and physiological processes involved is helpful to the practitioner, only a small part of it is really necessary.

What the confusion of knowledge and skills in medicine does accomplish is the intimidation of non-physicians, persuading them that they cannot play any serious role in the diagnostic and therapeutic processes. This characteristic is also true of other forms of education. Ivan Illich notes in his book, *Deschooling Society*:

The public is indoctrinated to believe that skills are valuable and reliable only if they are the result of formal schooling. The job market depends on making skills scarce and on keeping them scarce, either by proscribing their unauthorized use and transmission or by making things which can be operated and repaired only by those who have tools or information which are kept scarce. [6]

The labour power of physicians is a commodity. By keeping it scarce on the marketplace, they maximize their return on it. By obfuscating the relationship between skills and knowledge in medicine, medical education succeeds in making the necessary tools and information inaccessible to laymen.

As a result, other health workers and patients are not able to participate with physicians in the delivery of health care. They are bit players, while physicians stand at centre stage. But most medical situations do not require such an arrangement.

Talking about alienated social relations, Marx says: "[E]very person speculates on creating a new need in another, so as to drive him to a fresh sacrifice, to place him in a new dependence..." [7]

Physicians, through their own professional exclusivity, place others in a dependency relationship to their skills and knowledge. This benefits them economically and in other ways, often at the expense of others. The needs that motivate them to keep their skills in scarce supply are alienated needs; relationships to patients contingent upon professionalism are alienated relationships. Cluttering the brain with facts that rarely serve any purpose other than opening doors to participation in the professional role is alienated learning. "It is not the satisfaction of a need; it is merely a means to satisfy a need external to it."

Notes

page 74: In the economic sense, of course, medical students are neither impoverished nor exploited through their study activity. On other levels, however, their experience and that of workers are not dissimilar. Though students do not *become* alienated through their work activity (because they do not participate in the process of production), their work experience is very much alienated, woven as it is into the fabric of an alienated society.

page 78: So much more concerned is the physician with determining the cause of illness than its cure, that one hears not infrequently the astonishing admonition "a live patient with no diagnosis is better than a dead patient with a diagnosis" — so great is the desire to intervene even when the tests present a serious risk.

4

Doctors, Nurses
and Students

The Hospital Hierarchy

All relationships within a hospital are based on the authority of one person over another. When medical students first arrive on a hospital ward, they immediately find themselves enmeshed in a pre-existing, well-defined system of hierarchical work relations. Taking their place alongside (or more likely in back of) staff physicians, residents and interns, students join the medical sector of the ward community, which — apart from patients — otherwise consists almost exclusively of people whose work supports the doctors in their therapeutic activities. The most visible members of this "ancillary" staff are the nurses. But there is no doubt that the most powerful members of the hierarchy are the doctors.

Not only does this hierarchy define matters of authority and power, but it also provides an apparent limitation of contact between the different levels of worker. Albert Wessen, who did a study some time ago of communication between doctors, nurses and other health workers on the ward of a hospital, detailed what he called "an almost caste-like set of segregatory patterns".* The patterns, according to Wessen, "quite effectively limit informal interaction between hospital personnel of different ranks". Furthermore, he saw that the more "social distance" existing between occupational groupings, the less likely it would be for interaction to take place between those groupings. He concluded that there is "a well nigh universal tendency for those of high social rank to be freed from the obligation to interact with those of lower degree except on their own terms". And, as we shall see in this chapter, looking first at the stratified nature of life in a hospital and then at the structured relationships between the people working there, there has been little change in the system since Wessen did his study.

Perspectives on the hospital

The modern hospital is an institution established by one segment of society to provide acute medical care for that society. It is ruled by a board of directors, under the auspices of a government, a religious order or a private corporation. The structure of the hospital reflects certain presumptions about the proper organization of health care; it also reflects the degree to which the board has been influenced by various interest groups. The result is that the ill person's possibility of experiencing illness in a setting of his or her own choosing is almost certainly pre-empted.

My own earliest memory of a hospital visit is when, at the age of nine, I went to see my father who was incarcerated in the St. Boniface Hospital in Winnipeg after a heart attack. When I got to the hospital I was upset to learn that because of my age I would not be allowed to visit my father. Dismayed at the prospect of not seeing him for a long time, I decided to disobey the regulations. I trekked up several flights of stairs to his ward, only to be confronted by someone in authority — a nurse-nun — who scolded me and sent me back. I made up my mind there and then that hospitals were large, unfriendly places with lots of stairs, inhabited by people in strange costumes who were not nice to little boys. While my appreciation of the structure and organization of hospitals has been tempered by considerable experience since then, I still believe my judgement at age nine was quite close to the mark.

My next visit to a hospital occurred the summer before I entered medical school. When I was trying to make up my mind whether or not a medical career was for me, a distant relative in his final year of medicine at McGill took me on a whirlwind tour of the medical school buildings and of the hospital where he was working. No longer an unwelcome visitor, I expected to gain considerable insight into the workings of the hospital. I did not. Instead of obtaining a sense of the whole, I was left with a series of vague impressions.

The most striking of these was the 'antiseptic smell' so charac- teristic of hospitals. Although I had encountered that smell before, it made a deeper impression this time because I was carefully measur- ing the bouquet against the prospect of having to tolerate it for much of my future working life; I found the smell repulsive and nauseat- ing. Only much later did I develop the ability to recognize each of the dozens of commingling odours that played upon my nostrils that night. To anyone other than a hospital worker, they could only have smelled Hospital.

The hospital was dismal and depressing. We frequently en- countered unpleasant situations involving people who were physically or emotionally exposed in ways they certainly did not choose and probably would not have permitted had they been anywhere else. As we hustled down corridors, I was unable to retain a sense of proportion. I had no idea what part of the hospital I was in at any time. I had difficulty remembering what floor I was on. Only the interns' quarters seemed real. There I found situations I could relate to: a well-attended coffee percolator, people sitting around a television set, some reading the newspaper, most discussing something non-medical such as the baseball standings. Otherwise it was a journey through purgatory: dismal, depressing scene resolved into dismal, depressing scene. It was a disorienting experience even with an escort.

I was intimidated by the hospital and when I left that day, I certainly did not expect that I could ever enjoy spending much time in such a place. Of course, I did return to spend considerable time in several hospitals, and my perspective of that day has long since been superseded.

The corridors of illness
Each hospital has its peculiarities and idiosyncrasies, of course, but the differences in detail are rarely significant beside the very important similarities. Big and multifaceted, their characteristically demented architecture intimidates most outsiders, who have to ask frequent directions when trying to get about. Once a particular objective is attained, the visitor dares not wander too far astray but instead is grateful merely to have seen a perilous journey come to a satisfactory end. Effectively (albeit unintentionally) discouraged from learning more about the place than a particular situation or need requires, the visitor is limited to a unfortunately narrow perspective on the hospital.

In Montreal, one hospital is significantly more confusing than all the rest: the Royal Victoria Hospital, where I did my internship and junior residency, and in which I spent much time as an undergraduate as well. Had the planners set out to build a hospital more impenetrable to the average citizen than this one they could not have managed it. Were there a Nobel Prize for labyrinthine structures, the Royal Vic would win it regularly.*

Expeditions into this hospital are even more than usually demanding. Even after the front door is breached (it is easy enough to miss), visitors are by no means guaranteed immediate access to the particular facility they seek. For example, to reach the gynecology department, the intruder (in most cases female) must follow a long corridor to a statue of a rather stern Queen Victoria. There, a bank of elevators stands ready to carry her to the eighth floor, where she must debark. Next she must follow an even longer corridor to a fork where she must choose between a well lit, attractive corridor leading to the private ward and a dark, dismal one seeming to lead no- where but actually providing access to gynecology. If she makes the right choice and goes along this corridor far enough, our exhausted traveller may find herself in the *basement* of the Women's Pavilion, usually without realizing it or believing that she is there. If she then wishes to go to the gynecology clinic, she must have the presence of mind to find the one elevator (of three) going *down* from the base- ment to the clinic! If, instead, she wants to visit someone on the gynecology ward, she must ride up to the fifth floor where, more often than not, she will find herself separated from her friend's ward by the operating theatres. She must then go down a floor, over a bit and up again in order to reach her destination. Along the way, she will undoubtedly be scolded for having tried to pass through corridors that are closed to the public.

Other departments and their specialty clinics can be equally difficult to locate and to attain. Particularly challenging are the neurology and the psychiatry departments. Each is in a separate building virtually inaccessible from the front door of the hospital. The isolation of psychiatry takes on a concrete meaning in this in- stitution.

Most other hospitals are only a little easier to penetrate.* A visitor is unable to perceive any integration or systematization. If there is any unifying theme, it is the ubiquity of confusion, intimida- tion and obscurity.

Of course, hospitals are not designed on purpose to be that way. Most started out as much smaller edifices than they have be- come. The life history of any university hospital or large general hospital is one of piecemeal growth. Each element of the hospital community tends to seek expansion of its own domain: clinical de- partments want new specialty wards devoted to their field; scien- tists want expanded research facilities; conscientious medical educators want more teaching space within the hospital complex.

Rarely can a hospital remain one size for very long. In response to the demands of different interest groups within its walls, the available space is allocated, reallocated and supplemented in a haphazard way. The Royal Vic resembles a set of building blocks strung together in no particular order, each new one reflecting those interests most influential in the hospital at the time of construction, those able thereby to lobby more effectively than others for in- creased space.

The resultant confusion and intimidation of patients or visitors is inadvertent, but though no one conspires to make hospitals impenetrable, neither does anyone stop and say: "Let us plan and develop this place in as humane a way as possible."*

But visitors-intruders have other worries besides the fear of losing their way. A major difficulty for outsiders is that, whether lost or not, they are made to feel out of place by most hospital situations encountered. Walking down a corridor, they may be troubled by the thought that they have unknowingly wandered into a restricted area, a notion reinforced by stern glances from hospital workers (in whose way they always seem to be). While riding in an elevator they may be caught in a crossfire between physicians engaged in doctor talk or nursing assistants caught up in nursing-assistant talk, which may make them feel like eavesdroppers.

In the countless hospital situations in which ill, half-naked patients are exposed to passers-by, outsiders cannot help but feel at least a little out of place. Hospitals rarely have built-in privacy and discretion; on the rare occasions when they do, a distinction is made between their 'private' and their 'semi-private' or 'public' facilities.

In its organization as a workplace, as we shall see, the hospital fosters many distinctions and rigid functional differences among workers, for each group of whom 'hospital' means something quite different. But also built in is a distinction between hospital people and all others — the patients and visitors. Their perspective is that of outsiders, to the process of health care delivery as well as to the hospital itself. That they find the hospital overwhelming and confusing is but a consequence of this important fact of their relationship to the hospital and its work.

A staff stratified

The structure and organization of the hospital says a great deal about the attitudes and priorities of those who planned it. There is a special room for physicians to work in on each ward, and another for the nurses. There is an interns' lounge accessible to no one but the house staff. Each ward has a washroom for staff members only. Each group of workers has its own changing area. Some sections of the hospital — the private wards — are made to be much more comfortable and luxurious than others. Most of these particulars of hospital design reflect the assumption that there are classes of people who should not all be treated alike.

This is one manifestation of a phenomenon that is central to the organization of the hospital and often reflected in its architecture — the stratification of the work force.[1] Ostensibly based on levels of medical expertise, the stratification inevitably carries over into other spheres, creating a hierarchy that is social, cultural and economic as well as professional. Oddly enough, this stratification is most easily and comprehensively observable in the one place in the institution where medical considerations are irrelevant and access unrestricted— the cafeteria. Where you sit in the cafeteria depends very much on where you stand in the hierarchy.

For instance, at the Royal Victoria cafeteria a special section is cordoned off from the rest by potted plants: this is the preserve of the attending physicians (the specialists) who need not endure the sometimes harrowing line-up for food and can, instead, proceed directly to their private accommodations where they will be waited upon at set tables complete with tablecloths. And even when this smaller section is closed, most attending physicians can be seen sitting in that part of the main cafeteria closest to "their" area.

Other staff are scattered out in groups in the larger room, and each group tends to stick with its own. The housekeeping staff, some orderlies and occasionally a few nursing assistants sit in one row, close to the area where food is dispensed. In another area the residents, interns and fourth-year medical students sit together. There is another section where nurses, nursing assistants and technical staff sit, although even there they tend to keep their distance from each other. And then, near the entrance to the cafeteria there are two tables reserved for administrative personnel. These are the tables furthest from where the medical staff sit.

If this informal but well-defined seating arrangement is not enough, there is also the fact that every worker in the hospital wears a uniform that is a direct reflection of rank. Maintenance and house-keeping staff wear green uniforms; thus the first row of tables in the Royal Vic cafeteria is a sea of green. Other hospital workers, most of whom wear white, would appear almost to be soiling themselves were they to sit amongst people so obviously 'unclean'! These green-costumed workers are mostly recent immigrants; the social barriers between them and the rest of the staff merely reinforce the ethnic tensions and the linguistic barriers that also complicate interaction.

Nurses wear white. Nursing students are denied this honour, so they must settle for pink or blue outfits. Resident staff and senior medical students wear white shirts and pants. Junior medical students on some electives are also allowed to wear 'whites', an opportunity few pass up. Some senior residents emulate the attending physicians and wear long white coats. Administrative staff wear civilian clothes. Thus it is quite simple to tell just who is sitting where in the cafeteria. It is also obvious if anyone is "out of place". Even with no formal barriers or rules to restrict them to one part of the room, for each group of workers this room *is* the few tables at which they regularly sit. The status of the group determines the portion of the cafeteria that is real for them and, likewise, that portion of the hospital to which they relate and of which they are conscious.

Students and the "real world"

Medical students enter the hospital with much the same perspective as laypersons, but medical education alters their perception of their workplace and they soon begin to learn the way about. Thanks largely to membership in an elite group within the institution, they not only become familiar with the physical plant, but also increasingly acquire the capacity to feel comfortable in situations that would initially have been stressful.

First, they learn to feel at home in the interns' lounge, where they can go for a cup of coffee. Then the medical library becomes part of their psychic space. Next they become acclimatized to the wards, about which they strut self-assuredly. After that, they learn to feel at home in the radiology (x-ray) department. Then come the emergency room, the operating theatres and the clinics. Their confidence in belonging grows with each step.

Because students become insensitive to those aspects of the hospital that upset others, they are differentiated from the outsiders. To the extent that they can feel comfortable in most parts of the hospital, their perspective also differs from that of orderlies, cleaning staff and even many nurses who feel ill at ease when venturing into areas where they do not usually work.

Medical students learn how to move about the hospital most efficiently, learning shortcuts that are not apparent to visitors. Knowing their way around gives them a greater sense of the whole: they are able to integrate their experiences and be neither so overwhelmed nor so mystified as many others.

Some of this new-found perspective is shared with other hospital workers. Like them, students soon become oblivious to the continuing bombardment of their senses with the many faces of illness, a fact of hospital life which can be disorienting for the newcomer.

In the interns' quarters they have one relatively humane space that does *not* exist for most. Because this respite is available to them, they feel the degradation, dehumanization and depersonalization of hospital experience less acutely than the other workers who do not have this kind of private space to themselves.

Indeed, students hardly become aware at all of some aspects of the hospital that are of paramount importance to others. Visiting hours are one of the most important facts of hospital organization for patients and their guests; if they matter at all to physicians-in-training, it is only in the negative sense that visitors keep them from their work. There were many times when I worked on a ward and did not even find out, in all the time I was there, precisely what the visiting hours were. Similarly, the changing and lounge areas for non-medical staff are just as foreign to the medical student as the interns' quarters are to the orderly.

There is one more very important aspect to the changing perspective of the medical student to the hospital. When I toured the Montreal Children's Hospital the summer before I entered medical school, I felt sure I could never tolerate spending much time in such an institution. It was a relief to escape from that eerie, confusing, unfriendly, foreign and (in terms of my experience) *unreal* atmosphere.

But each subsequent year I spent more and more time Inside. Even before our introduction to clinical sciences, some of our lectures were given in hospital amphitheatres. Eventually, as I undertook clinical work, I began to spend more nights in the hospital and by the time I was interning I had very different feelings about being there. One day, early in my internship, after some sixty consecutive hours on duty, I wrote:

Upon emerging, I feel as though the world I am entering were unreal. So little of importance is happening out here: just people going about their mundane affairs. Behind me, I have left the hospital — so profound, so intense, so real. The hospital has become what is real for me; that is very disturbing.

This remarkable transformation in perspective was indeed disturbing. Physicians become so immersed in the 'reality' of the hospital that they may have considerable difficulty understanding how another person, a non-physician, perceives a shared situation. It makes it difficult to relate to those others.

Perspectives on the hospital tend to be determined by the roles people play in its inflexible organizational structure.* Medical students, as rather special travellers through the hospital, experience its environment through a progression of roles. In each role there are different economic, social and psychological relations to those around them, with the consequence that their perspective is continually changing. Yet the changes are quite predictable and mirror the students' socialization into the role and the outlook of the physician.

The shortcomings of hospitals that I have been discussing are in fact shortcomings of society. Hospitals are "alienated", to use Marx's term, because they reflect an alienated social order, an order characterized by domination, exploitation and lack of fulfillment.

For this fundamental reason, attempts to "humanize" hospital structures fail to humanize people's perceptions of and relations to this environment. The McMaster Medical Centre in Hamilton, Ontario, has an interior design that is aesthetically far more pleasant than most hospitals. As worthwhile as this may be, it does not eliminate, for instance, the intimidation that many patients and visitors feel when passing through its doors. Workers' perspectives, too, are independent of physical niceties. The recent painting of the cafeteria at the Royal Vic made it much prettier, but did not reduce the rigid stratification of the seating arrangements. In hospitals as elsewhere, alterations in the physical structure are of little significance if the social structure is left unchanged.

The physician hierarchy

Relationships between physicians, like all other relationships in a hospital, are very much a function of each doctor's own respective position. At first glance it may be difficult to discern a hierarchy within that amorphous mass of people called doctors. All of them wear white coats and stethoscopes and, along with their pipes, most sport that peculiar expression of self-confidence and studied superiority which, in the hospital, can be seen only on the faces of members of the medical profession. ("And how is my little leiomyosarcoma this morning?").

The fact that physicians do stand apart from everyone else in the hospital is enough alone to give the impression of solidarity. They hold a monopoly on patient care and decision-making. They attend conferences, examine patients and play diagnostic and therapeutic roles that are only occasionally accessible to other health workers, and almost never to patients.

Because of their rights and privileges, physicians are regarded as a class apart. Implicit in their attitudes and behaviour is the notion that the hospital exists only to provide them with a convenient forum for their ministrations to the sick. Everyone else is there to help out. Whenever I thought about my own position in the hospital subculture during my years of clinical training, it was almost always in relation to the physician community. I believe that I was not at all atypical in this respect.

In spite of their apparent uniformity, however, profound differences among them in rank and status divide the medical men and women of the hospital. The hierarchy ranges from the lowly first or second-year medical students fumbling through their first physical examination, to the chairman of a major clinical department with, perhaps, an international reputation. Between them are many gradations of knowledge, skill, and authority within the institution.

Attending physicians

The full-fledged specialists on a hospital's permanent staff are known as the **attending physicians**. They are not a homogeneous group. After years of slogging their way up the hierarchy of physicians-in-training, the newly certified subspecialists suddenly find themselves at the bottom of a whole new totem pole, still very much at the mercy of bosses. And the biggest bosses of all are the heads of the clinical departments.*

A department chairman, usually called "Chief", controls most major decisions in a department, including those involving salaries, space allocation, construction, hiring, firing, promotion and clinical and research priorities. Chiefs generally have unlimited tenure in the position. In short, they are autocrats.

Immediately below the department chairmen in the hierarchy are the Chiefs of Service, those lesser eminences responsible for the administration of the internal medicine wards. These people are truly the Chief's subordinates, in spite of their importance and seniority, because they lack an independent power base. Dependent upon the Chief for their positions and authority, most are also consistently loyal to the Chief's policies.

Equal in rank to the Chiefs of Service are the heads of the subspecialty divisions: the Cardiologist-in-Chief, the Nephrologist-in-Chief, the Gastroenterologist-in-Chief and so on. These people control the budgets in their respective divisions, and they are responsible for the organization and priorities of their subspecialties within the hospital. If they are big-time researchers, they *can* develop independent power bases. Subspecialty heads who can attract substantial outside funding can maintain their own direction and priorities, in spite of any disagreements with their Chief.

Most other physicians have two affiliations: to a subspecialty division and to a general medical ward or service. They are thereby subject to authority through two channels. At least in public, most faithfully toe the line. But even among these non-commissioned attending physicians, there are some differences in rank. The junior people are obliged to spend the greater part of their time working in community hospitals affiliated with the university centre. Senior physicians, on the other hand, rarely have to go out into the field.

The method of payment also reflects rank. Most senior physicians receive a full salary from the hospital. Some are allowed to earn a little extra on the side to supplement their salaries.* Junior attending physicians are usually given only a portion of their allowable income as salary. They are obliged to go out and work for the rest; if they don't make it, they don't get it. If they earn more in this way than allowed they must turn the surplus over to the hospital.

The junior person is very much a child in the department. These people often have inferior office space, less secretarial help and less convenient examining facilities. How bad a deal they get administratively usually depends on where they stand in the graces of the Chief.

Even worse off are the private practitioners. Some of them are allowed to send patients to the hospital for admission but not to care for them once inside. Others are allowed to visit and care for their patients in hospital, but only occasionally do they have an opportunity to "attend" on a ward (supervise the work of the resident staff).

Hail to the Chief

While the relative rank of attending physicians is expressed in different ways in different institutions, the absolute power of the Chief is consistently characteristic of clinical departments. In this respect, the difference between other departments of a university and those in the hospital is quite startling. Elsewhere in the university, a chairman of a department is generally considered to be the first among equals; in the hospital, the chairman is king of kings.

The chief of a major clinical department in one Montreal hospital, for instance, has held his job for two decades and seems to be permanently entrenched. His perpetuity is a cause for chagrin to many of the physicians on staff. Their discontent stems not from frustrated ambitions to take his place, but from a concern shared with the resident staff that he is providing totally unsatisfactory leadership. It is said that he has maintained his power through sophisticated political manoeuvrings, allocating positions of importance to his cronies, and nurturing good relations with the hospital's Board of Directors.

Another departmental chief was left behind by modern science many years ago. Nevertheless, he has preserved his power and has encountered little active opposition from the many bright young people in his department. Most of them recognize his inadequacy but swallow their pride and continue to pay him allegiance even as he imposes his outdated notions on their work. Rather than attempt to unseat him, they snipe occasionally behind his back and count aloud the days remaining until his obligatory retirement.

I spent some time at a hospital in the southern United States where the Physician-in-Chief does not just stand head and shoulders above his colleagues. He has quite literally placed himself upon a pedestal: there is a statue of him in the main lobby of the large municipal hospital he has dominated for a quarter of a century. Elsewhere in the building there is a small museum named for him. He is quite well known in his specialty throughout the United States, but apparently his ego is even bigger than his reputation.

Not all Chiefs are so firmly entrenched as to be invulnerable to overthrow. One who is clearly incompetent and out of step with departmental priorities can be dethroned, but it is unusual. The only Chief I ever came across who was deposed was being punished for an altogether different kind of offence. This man, who worked at a medical centre in California, had left-wing political views. During the period of campus unrest related to the war in Vietnam he became involved in a Faculty Political Action Group. Apparently, this was inappropriate conduct for the Physician-in-Chief of a university hospital. Even so, it took an administrative sleight of hand to have him turfed out. When a new dean was selected for the medical school, he received *pro forma* the resignations of all departmental chairmen, as was routine. For the first time in the school's history, the dean accepted a resignation so submitted — that of the activist.

The importance of a Chief to the department, its priorities, its tone and outlook, is remarkable. Departments of internal medicine in many hospitals in North America recently went through a period of crisis in which they were unable to fill their chairmanships with "suitable candidates". Some went months, or even longer, without a Chief, so crucial did they feel it was to select the right person. Most departments seem to prefer a "superstar" as Chief, a man who can attract outsiders and remake the department in His (not likely Her) own image.

The power of the Chief is of two types: real power, which is the authority to make decisions concerning the work and careers of colleagues, and pseudopower resulting from the fact that superior intellect and clinical skills are thought to be synonymous with the exalted office. Many Chiefs encourage others to treat them with excessive deference, but this pseudopower exists mostly in the minds of colleagues, reflecting their willingness to submit to the Chief's authority.

The Physician-in-Chief of one hospital likes to talk. Every time he goes to a hospital conference (typically, the weekly Medical Grand Rounds), he occupies several minutes of conference time summing up what he considers to be poignant and important in the case or topic under discussion. Unfortunately, he never has anything significant to say, and is rarely able to come up with anything even relevant. Nevertheless, he is able to command the right to speak because as Chief he is, of course, the wisest of all.

This instance illustrates what might be called **intellectual authoritarianism** in the hospital, which assesses the validity of a person's point of view or the reliability of clinical judgement in proportion to rank. Of course, the eminence of a particular physician in the discipline also counts. Without solid reputations, doctors may not receive the deference due their particular rank when they are obviously off base. Normally, however, it is only the deviants who are willing to express the belief that their Chiefs do not know what they are talking about.

The supposition that the top man's judgement is inevitably correct has been commented upon in the medical literature and described as the "emperor's clothes syndrome".[2] A typical scenario for this syndrome occurs at a hospital bedside, where a group of physicians (from medical student to Cardiologist-in-Chief) are examining a patient. The Big Man listens to the patient's heart after hearing a summary of the intern's findings. As he listens his brow furrows, and he remarks: "I can hear a fourth heart sound."

Now, none of the others heard this fourth heart sound but they are not about to argue. In turn they go over to the patient, place their cold stethoscopes on his chest, listen, and humbly indicate their concurrence. Only the student, if he or she has not been around long enough to know better, might come out with the opinion that there is no fourth heart sound to be heard.*

Intellectual authoritarianism is in the finest traditions of medicine. Galen, a second-century Greek physician, very dogmatically and incorrectly described human anatomy on the basis of his dissection of dogs. "See for yourself", Galen told his readers. They looked, repeating the dissections according to his protocol, and saw what he saw. Their perceptions were compromised by their preconceptions. It was not until some fifteen hundred years later, in the seventeenth century, that William Harvey destroyed Galen's system with his discovery of the circulation of blood and physicians came to realize just how wrong the great master had been.

But not all physicians submit to the intellectual authority of their superiors. One doctor, for example, makes his presence felt whenever his subspecialty holds a conference at McGill, by telling his Chief and all other physicians in the division that they are, so to speak, full of incorrect information and observation. He is a very bright fellow but almost universally disliked by his colleagues. I believe that their attitude stems from resentment at his nerve in speaking out while they do not. It is generally acknowledged that his propensity for letting others know what he thinks makes it unlikely that he will ever be promoted in the future.

The Chiefs are patriarchs. All but the most senior members of the departments they rule are known as their "Boys". When a physician joins the staff, the newcomer joins so-and-so's department; not surprisingly, it is difficult to remove a person who accumulates political capital in this way. The intrigues of departmental politics can only properly be considered in the light of the Chief's absolute pre-eminence.

Physicians-in-training

Below the attending physicians in the hospital hierarchy are the clinical fellows (subspecialty trainees), the house officers (residents and interns), and the medical students. This group — the **physicians-in-training** — is also highly stratified.

At the bottom rung are the medical students. Some are surprised to discover just how low they rank when they emerge from the subordination and frequent humiliation of the preclinical years, but they learn their place soon after arriving in the hospital. Ultimately they are able to inch up the steep slope towards the spectacular summit as they become third-year, then fourth-year students, interns, junior assistant residents, senior assistant residents, residents, chief residents and clinical fellows.

The relations among physicians-in-training at these many levels are closely tied to their relations with attending physicians. Many house officers are extremely deferential to the physicians they work under. While they do not hesitate to express contempt for some, they are uncritically admiring of others. For at least a few, this is an indication of the extent to which they have selected certain of their professors as role models.

One attending physician, a neurologist, told me that his residents frequently tried to emulate his own behaviour. "There was one resident whose inflections, gestures, mannerisms, everything, were in obvious imitation of me," he said. "It became rather embarrassing after a while." This sort of behaviour is most evident in surgical trainees, who consistently assimilate the grandiose and majestic presence of their patrons.

Unfortunately, the close identification of house officers with their physician superiors can have negative effects on patient care in any specialty. There is, for instance, an obvious example of this in the area of urology. Urologists, the surgical subspecialists who deal with the urinary tract and the male genital system, have a preponderance of elderly patients with problems of the prostate. Because of their age, these patients often have complicated courses and long convalescences. They also frequently have several other diseases at the same time. This makes them ideal candidates for dumping — discharge prematurely from the hospital or transfer to another ward on the pretence that their urological problems are no longer their major hindrance to discharge. In the latter instance, their diabetes or cough has suddenly become too big a problem for the urology ward to handle, even with the help of a visiting consultant.*

It is very much in the interest of attending urologists to get rid of these patients. It frees beds for other patients and permits the urologists to perform more operations and make more money. It is only marginally in the interest of the residents on a urology ward to play this game — they may gain a little additional experience but at the same time commit themselves to more work and certainly to ignoring the needs of the patient. But to a large degree these house officers have come to identify their own needs so closely with the needs of attending physicians that they are ready to sacrifice both their own and their patients' best interests to them.

It can, of course, work the other way. One night when I was working in Emergency, a woman with a particularly intriguing set of abdominal symptoms came in. The intern who saw her asked the medical resident-on-duty for his opinion as to the diagnosis. The resident too found the case a little difficult. I noticed that he examined the patient's urine and did a white cell count on her blood himself. He then wrote an extremely comprehensive note on the patient's chart. I asked him why he did all this, since the urinalysis and white cell count were the intern's responsibility, and the resident was not obliged to write more than a short note unless he disagreed with the intern's findings.

"Well," he explained, "she is Dr. Thinskin's patient. He's a tough bastard and it's two in the morning. I'm going to have to wake him up and tell him what I plan to do. If he asks me anything about her that I don't know, or if any of the lab data prove to be inaccurate, then he'll shit all over me. I don't want that to happen."

This kind of unnecessary subservience to senior physicians sometimes manifests itself as outright toadying — currying favour for whatever career or academic benefit it might bring. One resident of my acquaintance would spend most of his day watching for the arrival of this or that prominent attending physician on the ward. Before any of the rest of us would even be aware of the doctor's presence, this resident would have him buttonholed, arm around his shoulder, taking credit for whatever breakthroughs we had made since his last visit.*

If house officers often find themselves grovelling before the grown-ups, it is not always at their own initiative. During my first week on a ward during third-year medical school a classmate and I decided, at the suggestion of our tutor, to attend the weekly ward conference. We got to the conference room ten minutes early, the first to arrive. Finding two rows of empty chairs, we sat down in the front row. But when the Chief of Service came in a few minutes later, he came over to tell us, "Of course boys, you are welcome at these sessions, but you must sit in the second row."

By such experience you quickly learn your place in the hierarchy. For some, the initiation was worse than for others. One group of students in third year had to present a case to the Chief of Service in one of the hospitals they were rotating through. It was a traumatic and abhorrent ordeal for all of them. The Professor invariably took to task students who were presenting cases, picking holes in presentations, often on trivial points, and following up by grinding the students in the ground, leaving them profoundly humiliated.

Some of our teachers were overtly sadistic, others were not. But given the context of our encounters, even with the latter their dominance and our submissiveness was inevitable. After all, the teachers were perpetually evaluating our knowledge and performance. In third-year medical school, it seemed the key to our continuing success lay in the oral examinations and case presentations. These were not only important in the determination of our grades but also in the teachers' development of the subjective impressions that would be crucial later on if we wanted letters of recommendation.

Frequently, especially in third year, our performance was assessed by professors who hardly knew our names. First impressions, which were often the only impressions, could be decisive and we had to be on our toes at all times. On one occasion a classmate of mine presented a case to our clinical supervisor while we sat in a small dining area in the intern's quarters. Part way through his presentation, a muskrat wandered up to the window— a rather unusual sight in downtown Montreal. All of us, including our teacher, went over to the window to watch the animal while the presentation continued.

After the student had finished, the Man, who had hardly listened and was still looking out of the window, casually remarked: "You really weren't very well organized."

Although it was not true, that judgement cast the student permanently in the professor's bad graces. One day some time later the same teacher asked if any of us would be willing to give blood for an experiment he was doing. My maligned colleague volunteered enthusiastically. Afterwards he confided, "I'll give all the blood I've got..." But his efforts were to no avail. He still received the anticipated and undeserved poor grade.

Since so many of our encounters with attending physicians could potentially bear such fruits, our relationships with these people were inevitably structured and stilted. The amount of say that anyone has in determining a grade is usually directly proportional to rank and inversely proportional to the amount of time spent with the student. At one evaluation session I attended as a resident, an attending physician turned to the house staff present and said, "Let's hear first from the the most important people — the residents." It was good to be recognized: in fact, we residents did know the students best. But in any case the attending physicians proceeded to ignore our judgements except when they coincided with their own.

Like physicians at other levels, house officers also discover very quickly that intellectual authoritarianism emphasizes their lowly position in the hierarchy. Once a group of us were discussing a case with a professor. The patient had hypoglycemia — low blood sugar — and the student presenting the case proposed that an insulinoma — a tumour in the pancreas — might be the cause. The professor squawked with dismay at this suggestion.

"Do you know how rare insulinomas are? There have been only 13 reported in the world literature. I have had the privilege of seeing three of these cases, all on different continents, in the same year."

Now, in this instance the professor was clearly mistaken. Insulinomas are not very common but neither are they quite that rare — I have seen three cases myself.* At the time, I did not believe for one minute what the professor was saying. Nor, as I later learned, did any of my colleagues. But none of us contradicted him. It did no one any good to have this man wandering around spouting misinformation, but none of us dared to speak out because he was, after all, the Professor. And, unfortunately, this intellectual authority of physicians can extend well beyond the bounds of their professional competence. The students come to feel that they must immerse themselves in their studies and learn a great deal before anything they say can be taken seriously, whether it be in relation to the principles of internal medicine, the lifestyle of the physician, the priorities of the health care system or the organization of society.

This kind of submission can play an important role in socializing medical students. Whatever capacity physicians-in-training still possess for independent thought will surely diminish as they submerge further into their medical identity and develop into replicas of those around them. "You will eat, drink, breathe and sleep medicine twenty-four hours a day for the rest of your lives," one professor told us and, out of eighteen students, only one objected. The rest of us looked on in astonishment, not at the professor's remark, but at the rebel's temerity.

Intellectual authority can sometimes assume the guise of moral authority. A Gynecologist-in-Chief I knew at one hospital was able to impose his morals on the whole department. Because he felt that abortion is murder, he would not co-operate in bringing the spirit of the 'liberalized' Canadian abortion law to bear on his department's policy. While a smaller hospital was doing hundreds of abortions each year, he was able to keep his hospital's tally below two dozen. Although there were many who did not share his attitudes, no one questioned his right to impose his will, with the exception of a group of women who staged a sit-in one year with the support of a few medical students.

Even when their interests in relation to a particular issue are clearcut, the resident staff is usually reluctant to take a stand that might arouse the ire of superiors. The extra hours we worked, going way beyond our contract agreement, were a case in point (see chapter two, pages 33-34). One intern, a refugee from a right-wing totalitarian state, expressed disgust at the timidity of the house staff. "Here, they don't need to use fascist tactics to get the workers to submit to abuses," he said.

The house staff hierarchy

The physician hierarchy is no less rigid in its lower than in its upper echelons. At each level of progress trainees are obliged to work a little less hard at mundane tasks (the dreaded 'scut' work), allowed to take on a little more responsibility and accorded a little more respect by those above and below in the hierarchy. Although this progression correlates somewhat with increasing competence, it is really a function of increasing status.

The most painful expression of the house staff hierarchy is found in those training programs with a 'pyramid system', a system where fewer positions become available at each step upwards in the hierarchy. I visited one medical centre in southern California just after a pyramid system had been introduced there. Several interns were openly furious about the way in which they had been dropped — they had not been aware when the year began that their numbers would be whittled away. Nevertheless, the fact that they were dropped without warning seems merciful compared with the situation in hospitals where trainees know all year long that not all will be kept on. In such instances, the competition for the coveted positions can be cutthroat.

In his book *The Making of a Surgeon* William Nolen has few reservations about the pyramid system at New York's Bellevue Hospital:

We started with seven interns on general surgery, and five years later, one would become chief resident. The pyramid was narrowed by several methods ... Some of the starters would be fired. If the guy was a goof-off, this wasn't too painful; but if he was a nice fellow who just wasn't quite as good as the man with whom he was competing, it was sad.[3]

Nolen's view, an optimistic one, is that the correct decision is inevitably made in the weeding-out process. This presumes, of course, that a competitor could not be trampled upon or out-manoeuvred by someone "who just wasn't quite as good". This is, after all, the perspective of a man who himself won out in the end. He expresses unreserved confidence in the ability of his own Surgeon-in-Chief to make the appropriate decisions about who should get the axe: "He [Dr. Stevens] could learn enough in five minutes to decide if the man was worth keeping for five years."[4] Not surprisingly, Nolen also accepted the notion that medical knowledge and competence are inevitably tied to rank:

You could tell when you became first assistant resident because suddenly there were more people asking you what to do than telling you what to do ...

I took Charlie aside and explained to him that as an A.R. (Assistant Resident) I naturally knew more about both the clap and appendicitis than he (an intern) did.[5]

In time, Nolen came to crave the "throne" of chief resident for himself:

The day that Dr. Stevens called me into his office and told me I was to be the next chief resident ranks with the day I received my acceptance at medical school, and if my wife will excuse me, my wedding day in my personal list of great moments.

In our pyramidal system with seven interns, twenty or so assistant residents, and only one chief resident, those who wanted the job lived in a perpetual state of anxiety: Will I ever get to be chief resident? The question wasn't always foremost in our minds, but it was there all the time. Now I had the answer — the job was mine. I felt ten feet tall.[6]

Doubtless, Nolen would have become a surgeon even if he had not been appointed chief resident. But his writing reveals an obsession with power and a concern for position and advancement in the hierarchy, unfortunately all too typical. Sometimes this kind of obsession can lead to considerable tension.

On one occasion when I was a student, the chief resident and the senior resident on my ward were both going away for a couple of weeks. They were leaving behind two medical students, an intern and a junior assistant resident who was to arrive the day after the other two departed. Before leaving, the chief resident designated the intern to run the ward in his absence, or so the intern claimed. When the junior resident arrived, the intern began to tell him what to do. In the hospital, this is far from the usual scheme of things, so religiously is rank respected. The friction between the two was obvious to all, and I, for one, felt very uncomfortable in the crossfire. The resident was in anguish throughout the two weeks; the intern revelled in the authority which he would not soon have an opportunity to exercise again. Most significant in this incident was that it mattered so much to all concerned what their particular status was.

Rank was important because it brought with it the authority that enabled them to dominate colleagues and others. As with Dr. Nolen, it assumed an importance out of all proportion to reality. How far removed can such concerns become from patient care and medical education!

Fledgling house officers are regularly trod upon by others, generally without justification. Not surprisingly, they develop an all-consuming passion to mount the hierarchy as rapidly as possible (and it can never happen quickly enough) in order to attain the respect of others, which has been consistently denied, to assume the responsibility that is perceived as a measure of maturity and to dominate those who have not yet climbed so far.

I doubt if many medical students realize, when they are starting out, just how little authority they will possess (or respect they will command) until they have reached the upper rungs of the professional ladder. If they did, few would be willing to continue tolerating the humiliations experienced at each stage.*

Competition within the hierarchy

The atmosphere promoted by the social organization of the physician community in the hospital is one into which destructive competitiveness is readily injected. Among medical students it is most typically expressed by the unsubtle lobbying for 'choice' internships in prestigious hospitals.

The number of sought-after internships has hardly changed in the last decade or two while the number of students pursuing them, particularly in internal medicine, has increased dramatically. Recognizing that they need to demonstrate some special talent or proclivity, many students spend much of their time trying to out-manoeuvre one another in the race for a place.

Competitiveness is endemic among trainees at all levels. On internal medicine wards it may be expressed as an attempt to out-shine one another in ward discussions and conferences. Surgical residents scramble for the status which, they feel, derives from the amount of 'cutting' they are allowed to do. One resident I knew made it a point to arrive in the operating room well before his attending surgeon, so that he could 'prep' and drape the patient and assume a position next to the sleeping body, scalpel in hand, in the hope that the surgeon would, as a result, be more inclined to let him operate.

Much of this competitiveness is petty but like the striving of so many physicians-in-training to dominate others or submit before authority, it is the norm. In an order as restrictive, autocratic and irrationally oppressive as the hospital medical hierarchy, the acceptance of hierarchical relations and the ritualization of progress through that hierarchy helps to make sense of what would otherwise be a frustrating, even unbearable situation. To the extent that accepting structured interpersonal relations with others makes life in the hospital tolerable for house officers, the hierarchy serves to socialize them into their role as physicians and into their 'professional' consciousness.

It is indeed unfortunate that physicians and physicians-in-training in the hospital are so entangled in authoritarian relationships that patient care can become a secondary consideration. It is beyond the scope of this book to deal with the quality of medical care, but, as I have intimated in various places, patient care may well suffer when the patient is incidental to the real work of physicians-in-training: rising through the ranks of their profession.

Working with nurses

Nurses do rank above other ancillary workers in the hospital hierarchy. But compared to physicians, their authority is small and their decision-making power trivial, no matter how experienced or capable they may be. In North American medicine there is no mechanism whereby nurses can upgrade their qualifications and become doctors.* Their only avenue for advancement lies within the ranks of their own profession and this cannot offer greater involvement in therapy or release them from subservience to physicians.

For subservience is unmistakably their lot. Endowed with little responsibility and authorized to make only the most limited kinds of decisions, nurses are required in all instances to follow the instructions of physicians. This is true even when the 'physicians' are utterly inexperienced medical students doing their first stint in a hospital. The resentment that this situation inspires is amplified by the rapid ascent of fledgling physicians to ever greater heights of power and professional responsibility.

During my year of internship there was a period of two months when I rotated, along with seven others, to the Emergency Room. Working in Emergency is one of the most important experiences in physician training, because it gives students their first opportunity to handle acute, life-threatening problems. So I was not alone in feeling insecure about my ability to make the appropriate decisions whenever necessary. Fortunately, the nurses who worked in the Emergency Department were generally very competent and used to assuming more responsibility than their colleagues elsewhere in the hospital. In many matters of judgement, they were far in advance of the bright-eyed interns, at least at first, and they knew it. When my group of interns arrived, a few of the nurses went out of their way to let us know, in quite sarcastic tones, just what they thought of our admittedly shaky judgement.

Their initial resentment was compounded if one of us made a decision that caused them unnecessary additional work; this often happened because we tended at first to err on the side of caution. I discovered this, rather painfully, on one of my first duty shifts in Emergency.

A young woman came to the hospital and told us that she had taken twelve pills of a certain medication. Part of the recommended treatment for an overdose of that medication is to pass a tube through the nose and into the stomach. Activated charcoal resin is sent down the tube and the treatment absorbs any of the drug that remains undigested in the stomach. Unfortunately, having had no experience with overdoses of anything other than aspirin, I was not aware that a dozen of these particular pills cannot harm an adult, and I asked a nurse to prepare the resin while I set about to pass the tube.

The nurse became very angry. "That's ridiculous," she scolded

me in a voice loud enough for everyone in the Emergency Department to hear. "Twelve of those pills is not an overdose. Can't you
see I'm busy? You're giving me extra work for nothing. Don't you
know *anything* about overdoses?"

After that tirade I felt about eighteen inches tall. A few minutes
later, after checking the toxic dose in a book and finding out she was
right, I told her not to bother. By this time, though, she had finished
preparing the charcoal and was even angrier.

Such incidents, though not commonplace, contribute to the
well-worn stereotype of the domineering and oppressive nurse
whose greatest delight consists in devising new ways to victimize
innocent medical students and interns.[7] And it is true that some
nurses can be formidable.* However, their behaviour can be understood only in its context: a work situation offering few responsibilities greater than the tedious "scut work" — drawing blood,
starting intravenous infusions, doing electrocardiograms — that
even novice physicians like to avoid.

The attitude of most medical students does nothing to make the
nurse's position less frustrating. As one nurse put it:

[A] few medical students just seem to be with it, they are able to understand
what you are trying to tell them, they are a pleasure to work with; most,
however, pretend to know everything and refuse to listen to anything we
have to say and I guess we give them a rough time.[8]

But initially it is only because students are relatively powerless
that nurses can behave with such impunity and so aggressively
towards them. As students progress through their education, they
encounter fewer and fewer instances where nurses assume temporary dominance over them. And, by the time they emerge as full-
fledged practitioners, they confidently dismiss all such displays of
resentment as manifestations of sexual frustration on the part of the
nurses concerned. Indeed, if they have been properly imbued with
the attitudes of their profession, they probably come to regard most
nurses as rather unintelligent menials with little to offer in the lofty
intellectual spheres that physicians are privileged to inhabit.[9]

So little do nurses count in the world of medical students and
interns that physicians often do not even remember the names of
many of the nurses they work with, though they probably do not
suffer from that problem when it comes to their fellow physicians
(this was certainly true of me). Nor will doctors often be aware of a
nurse's individual rank or qualifications. Some nurses have doctorate
or master's degrees; others have bachelor's degrees; still others are
registered nurses who would prefer not to be confused with the

licensed practical nurses and nurse's aides. In the context of the hospital hierarchy, many nurses feel degraded when they are taken for someone of "lower" rank. But physicians, preoccupied though they are with reckoning minute gradations of status within their own profession, often do not trouble to differentiate one nurse from another. It is not surprising that many nurses regard such indifference as an affront both personal and professional.

The patronizing attitude of physicians towards nurses comes through very clearly when medical questions are discussed on the ward. Even the lowliest medical students are encouraged to participate in these discussions, which are a vital part of their education.* Only infrequently, however, will nurses be invited to comment on a patient's condition, and for them to offer unsolicited opinions is unusual enough to be considered a reckless breach of ward protocol. This exclusion is hard to rationalize on any medical grounds, because nurses are much more in touch with patients than physicians can ever be, and hence are often in a position to make valuable contributions to therapeutic decisions.

Nor is this the only situation in which the authority structure of the hospital irrationally impedes the delivery of care. A specific instance of the irrationality as well as inefficiency of the system in this regard was related to me by an emergency room nurse. A staff physician was the only one covering the emergency room on a night when someone was brought in with acute pulmonary oedema, a condition in which the lungs are filled up with fluid, usually due to weakness of the heart. The physician-on-duty happened to be out of the emergency department when the patient was brought in.

Pulmonary oedema is a medical emergency. A patient who does not receive prompt treatment can die very quickly. Proper treatment includes administration of oxygen, application of tourniquets to the limbs (to stop the return flow of blood to the heart and lungs) and sitting the patient in an upright position. Certain medications must also be administered to reduce the workload of the heart.

The nurses recognized the patient's problem instantly. They paged the physician and gave the appropriate supportive care, but they could not give the medications until the doctor came. For ten crucial minutes, the physician did not appear, despite frantic and continued paging throughout the hospital. With the patient seated upright, tourniquets applied and oxygen flowing, the nurses could do little else. They started an intravenous infusion of sugar water so that medications could be administered. They drew up the required medications in appropriate dosages into syringes and stood poised by the patient's bedside. When the physician finally sauntered in, he gave the necessary permission for the potentially life-saving injections.

On this occasion the patient might have died because the rigid hospital hierarchy did not allow nurses to administer treatment on their own, even when they had the competence and experience to do so and even when, as in this case, there was no one else around to do it.*

In the face of the many frustrations inherent in their position, it is perhaps surprising that open expressions of resentment on the part of nurses are not more common. Yet while some nurses — particularly those with supervisory authority — are anything but submissive in their day-to-day demeanour, most act towards physicians with the utmost deference.

One nurse I encountered during my internship was so deferential, so compulsively subservient before physicians that she could be counted upon to say "Yes, Doctor" to any statement they might make. A few times I asked her to address me by my first name. "Yes, Doctor," was her invariable reply. This nurse's behaviour was obviously extreme. Yet submissiveness to physicians is the rule rather than the exception among nurses, and many subordinate themselves even more than necessary by declining extra responsibilities if they are offered.

Sometimes behaviour that is superficially submissive is in reality motivated by the need for greater responsibility, according to the rules of what Leonard Stein calls the "doctor-nurse game":

The nurse is to be bold, have initiative, and be responsible for making significant recommendations, while at the same time she must appear passive. This must be done in such a manner so as to make her recommendations appear to be initiated by the physician.[10]

In other words, nurses must play by the rules. If they do not underplay their recommendations as expected, they are characterized as overaggressive or, if they do not make any recommendations at all, as dullards. (Of course, this same pattern characterizes many male-female interactions in settings other than the hospital.) On the other hand, medical students or physicians who do not play along by accepting nurses' recommendations can be penalized, either by being treated aggressively or by being denied such traditional shortcuts as giving orders over the telephone.

The only other means whereby nurses can acquire extra responsibility is by advancing through the ranks of their colleagues. Nursing libraries are now well stocked with journals and books with titles like *Supervisor Nurse, Nursing Management,* or *Ward Administration.* A very common adaptation for nurses who cannot gain access to the power and status of a physician is to vie for positions of dominance over other hospital workers.

Two groups of people over whom nurses do wield authority are the orderlies and the nurse's aides. These workers are near the bottom of the hospital pecking order, the natural targets for the aggression of frustrated or humiliated nurses. One orderly gave me his opinion about how readily the nurses adopted the dominant role:

"All day long, the patients shit, piss and vomit on me. Twice a day at least the nurses shit on me too. When they ask me to do something, they *never* do it nicely. They are always letting me know who is boss. I can take it pretty well, but a lot of the guys can't. Quite a few of the orderlies are married immigrants from countries where sex roles are even more defined than here. They know better than to talk back to the nurses, but they're very resentful of the way they're treated by them."

Compensatory mechanisms of this kind, however, arising as they do from the exploitation of rank, cannot free nurses or other hospital personnel from the inescapable relationships of authority within the hospital. Nowhere is this brought home more vividly than in the operating room. Relations among personnel in the "O.R." are rigidly defined by status, even more than in other parts of the hospital. The person at the pinnacle of the operating room hierarchy is, of course, the surgeon. As William Nolen explains in *The Making of a Surgeon*:

The surgeon is the boss... The surgeon decides where to make the cut, what operation to perform, how to close the incision. He may ask his assistant for an opinion, but the ultimate decision is the surgeon's alone.[11]

Although Nolen does not point it out, the authority of surgeons extends well beyond operations themselves. To begin with, physicians are assisted into their operating garb in order of rank, with the surgeon first and the resident second. If medical students are present, they have extra time to scrub while waiting for gown and gloves.

During an operation, discussion is not always centred on the task at hand, since much of what has to be done is quite routine. Consequently, there is a great deal of banter about the previous night's football score or the sexual attractiveness of some nurse or patient. Such conversations are usually initiated by the surgeons. They set the tone for the conversation and contributions to the discussion are usually proportional to rank. Because of this, nurses make no contribution at all — it is not done. They are present at the operation in one of two capacities: either as a scrub nurse, who passes instruments on to the surgeon, or as a circulating nurse, who obtains any necessary instruments or equipment and passes them to the scrub nurse. These are very important roles in the operating room, as any surgeon will readily acknowledge: "Every operation is a team event. A surgeon can no more operate on a patient by himself than a general can fight a war alone. An operation, like a battle, is a cooperative venture."[12]

William Nolen's comparison of the operating room team to an army is apt, for the relationship of a surgeon to "his" nurses is comparable to that of a general to his footsoldiers: surgeons only communicate with nurses to give them orders. It is not particularly surprising, then, that in the chapter of his book devoted to the "O.R. team", Nolen was unable to talk about nurses for much more than two pages.

"Forceps... scalpel... suture... clamp..." This is the extent of nurse participation in the "team". It is hardly surprising that even on the occasions when nurses are asked their views on whatever is being discussed they are usually quite reserved in their responses. It is not their place to get involved in the discussion, because even conversation in the operating room manifests the hierarchy of the hospital.

The opportunities of nurses to behave aggressively in this situation are clearly limited, but in some circumstances openings do exist. My first experience in an operating theatre occurred when I spent an elective period working with heart surgeons in a California hospital. As third or fourth assistant in a coronary artery bypass operation (involving a vein graft from the leg to the chest) I was usually left to stitch up the leg after the vein had been removed. Invariably, I forgot what size of suture I was supposed to use and frequently I broke the needle by placing too much stress upon it. The nurse would clout me with a verbal sledgehammer every time this happened, usually making the blow that much more painful by sarcastically addressing me as "Doctor".

This particular nurse was again displaying the dual nature of the authority-oriented relationships that pervade hospital life. Guided by the authority structure, some contexts will inspire aggressive, and others submissive behaviour. Egalitarian behaviour between hierarchical planes is rare, and can only occur when the authority structure is either ignored or misunderstood by the parties involved.

This dual nature seems in itself to provide a clear refutation of a hypothesis presented by Leonard Stein in *The Doctor-Nurse Game* to explain the origins of authority-oriented behaviour in the hospital. The arrogant behaviour of physicians towards nurses, Stein says, is rooted in medical education, where medical students acquire an overwhelming fear of making a mistake. This becomes a phobia for the student, and "the classical way in which phobias are managed is to avoid the source of the fear." In order to accomplish this,

the physician develops the belief that he is omnipotent and omniscient, and therefore incapable of making mistakes . . . The slightest mistake inflicts a large narcissistic wound . . . Accepting advice from non-physicians is highly threatening to his omnipotence . . .[13]

Similarly, Stein argues that the tendency to submissiveness in nurses is the fault of nursing schools that "inculcate subservience and inhibit deviancy". It is certainly true that nursing schools have tended to encourage their students to submit gracefully before the physician (even, until recently, to the point of standing up when a physician entered the room).[14]

But since physicians are often *submissive* in their behaviour and nurses *domineering*, a better explanation is clearly called for. Such an alternative is the model of the authoritarian personality type, characterized by strivings for relationships based upon authority, either of the individual over others, or of others over the individual. This formulation can better explain much of the behaviour of physicians and nurses, both towards each other and towards others with whom they come into contact. I explore this concept in more detail later in the book.

There is one other aspect of the nursing situation we have not so far explored: the division of the sexes on occupational lines. How much of the friction between physicians and nurses, and between orderlies and nurses, arises from the fact that while orderlies and most physicians are men, virtually all nurses are women?

One need not look far to locate specifically sexist elements in the general pattern of oppression experienced by nurses. Just as many other working women are subject to the abuse of men holding more powerful positions, nurses are frequently victimized by the sexual chauvinism of physicians. Sexism can be open and blatant: Is she pretty? Is she married? Is she easy? That nurses want to be treated as sexual objects is a myth that has been perpetuated partly through the "literature" genre of nurse-novels.[15] It is also partly due to sex stereotypes that physicians tend to regard nurses as generally dull or unintelligent, and on this false basis exclude them from participation in medical deliberations.

It would be difficult to argue, however, that even the added burden of sexism makes the oppression of the nurse greater than that of the orderly or the nurse's aide, neither of whom is any stranger to the inflexibility of the authority structure of the hospital. Especially in their dealings with nurses, this structure is often painfully apparent.[16] Vincente Navarro argues that the problems of women working in health care cannot be isolated from the social and economic context:

[T]he so-called women's problem is the problem of men and society. Thus, to understand the situation of women in the health sector the distribution of political and economic power in the world of men must be studied... Just as poverty cannot be understood without an understanding of wealth, the distribution of wealth and the reasons for wealth and the income differentials in this country, the situation of women in the health sector cannot be understood without an understanding of the world of men and the distribution of social and economic power within that world. To understand the situation of women, then, one must analyse not women as such, but the entire socio-economic and political system that perpetuates the situation of women.[17]

Navarro identifies three major groupings within the economy: a **monopolistic sector**, which includes the manufacturing, insurance and banking industries; a **competitive sector**, which consists of trade and services; and a **state or public sector**, part of which contracts with the monopolistic sector in the provision of goods and services (such as the defence industry), and the other subsector of which provides services (such as health care).[18]

In this analysis, workers in the monopolistic sector are predominantly male, unionized and well paid. Workers in the competitive sector and in the service subsector are predominantly female, non-unionized and poorly paid.

In the health industry the upper-middle class (the physicians) is predominantly male. The lower-middle class (nurses, social workers and physiotherapists) is predominantly female, as is the working class, which comprises the majority of health workers (and includes dietary staff, cleaning personnel, nurse's aides, etc.)

As pointed out in chapter two, North American medical schools are now gradually beginning to admit more women students. This trend, praiseworthy in itself, is not likely to lead to the emancipation of other women who work in the area of health care. Those who do attain the status of physician are not particularly inclined to help their "sisters in struggle" who come from lower socio-economic groups. One group of women health workers expressed this very clearly:

The way doctors treat other female doctors, nurses, technicians, maids and dietary workers is clearly an oppression of women. But it is an oppression of women combined with class oppression. Most of us are college-educated women, regardless of our rank in our hospitals. We have trouble relating to young working class men who handle transportation and do maintenance work...

The 'aunt Tomasina' syndrome seems to be in evidence, in which women students and interns seem busily trying to improve themselves in a man's world by asserting their authority over everyone else, especially other women. Women who work with them are caught in the difficult trap of trying to treat an oppressor as a 'sister in struggle'.[19]

Comparing this type of experience with that of women in other spheres, Navarro suggests:

[T]he much needed improvement and correction of unfair policies affecting upper-middle class women in the health sector does not necessarily imply and is not necessarily followed by the betterment and the more urgent need of betterment of the lives of the majority of women in the health sector, the lower-middle class and the working class.[20]

Why do women occupy, for the most part, working class and some middle class positions in the work force? Navarro suggests that the division of labour, in which the family is a major determinant, is largely responsible. The relegation of women to unpaid housework and family raising allows employers to increase their profits: they only have to pay husbands (who are designated 'the providers'), thereby paying "for the work of one and [getting] the work of two".[21] Thus the division of labour within a household allows its members to be exploited. Furthermore, the exploitation is exacerbated by the use of women as a reserve army, able to supply labour in times of shortage. The positions in the work force made available in this way are inevitably underpaying and exploitative. The value system — sexism — which has grown along with this economic order ensures that women working in the health industry will be assigned a dependent role as appendages to the physicians and will accept this role as being appropriate:

Given these social and economic needs of the system, it is quite logical that women tend to be the majority of workers whose main function within the economy is to provide care and maintenance of the population, and that, within that sector, women tend to perform the conditional and dependent jobs.[22]

Sexual discrimination within the health labour force is not new. For centuries, women healers have been persecuted, sometimes as witches, for practising forms of healing that were not approved or merely for practising the recognized healing arts, as in the Paris trial of Jacoba Felicie in 1322.[23]

It was only a century ago, when Florence Nightingale took the Crimean War by storm, that the notion of women as ancillary or paramedical workers, subservient to the physician and dominant over 'lesser' workers, became acceptable to very many women.[24] Indeed, the very use of the term 'ancillary', from the Latin *ancilla*, a maid-servant, carries a double-edged implication of exploitation and sexism.[25]

"Class loyalties," observes Navarro, "are far stronger than sex loyalties."[26] As long as class divisions in the health labour force exist, we might anticipate that efforts to improve the status of women within the medical profession, though certainly needed, will be of little relevance to the great majority of women working in the health care industry.

Nor, until class differences have been eradicated, will the bizarre, unhealthy relationships resulting from the irrational allocation of authority finally cease to impede the delivery and sane practice of health care in our society.

Notes

page 81: During the period of Wessen's observations of communication on the ward of a hospital, 74 per cent of the communications of physicians were with other physicians, 23 per cent were with nurses and less than three per cent were with other health workers. Sixty-one per cent of nurse interactions were with other nurses, nine per cent were with physicians and 29 per cent were with other health workers. Only one per cent of the communications of other health workers were with physicians, 37 per cent were with nurses, and the rest were amongst themselves. (See A. Wessen, "Hospital ideology and communication between ward personnel", in W.R. Scott, E.H. Volkart [eds.], *Medical Care* [New York: John Wiley and Sons, 1966], pp466-467.)

page 83: From the outside, it looks like a medieval castle. This reflects a school of hospital design popular at the turn of the century when the Royal Vic was built. Across Pine Avenue from the hospital is Montreal's main water reservoir, providing at least a symbolic moat.

page 84: The outpatient department in Charity Hospital, New Orleans, is even worse. That amazing place is shared by two medical schools whose idea of working together is reminiscent of John Foster Dulles' partition diplomacy. Not only do these schools have separate wards, but also separate emergency and clinic areas on opposite sides of the building. A patient who did not know the ropes could sit outside a clinic whose label corresponded to the subspecialty indicated on his or her appointment slip only to discover (some hours later) that he or she "belonged" to the other medical school. I saw this happen to one woman who only discovered her error when it was too late for her appointment. The hospital was built as two large wings to allow the segregation of white patients to one side and blacks to the other — an arrangement that persisted until the early 1960s.

The UCLA Medical Centre in Los Angeles, where I completed my residency, and which boasts of being the world's second largest building (in square footage) after the Pentagon, has successfully confounded visitors for years; its principal access is through a hard-to-find "Temporary Main Entrance".

page 85: Needless to say, the workers who are engaged to construct a hospital have no opportunity to exercise creativity or spontaneity in their task. There is no opportunity for them to display initiative in the planning or execution, by drawing on their experience and assessment of what they and their families would like to see in the hospital. They are there, quite reasonably, to earn a living but in this objectification of their labour their potential for creative contribution is expropriated by those with the power to build the hospital (people who do not place high priority on the needs of the workers or others as consumers), no less than their labour power is expropriated by contractors (whose interest in the endeavour is to earn a profit).

page 88: Role-determined perceptions of the environment are quite common throughout society. Marx said that in modern society all of the relationships of people, all the objects they make, and all the structures they erect are reflections of their interaction with the existing socio-economic order. Every person is defined by who he or she is and what he or she does in a particular social and economic context. Relationships are a function of that definition. Subjective perceptions of objective reality express one's *utility* to the socio-economic order and are thereby alienated perceptions.

The perceptions people have in hospitals are warped by a restriction to the narrow, arbitrary roles of orderly, medical student, nurse, patient or visitor. Denied the opportunity to relate as whole persons to their work, to what they produce and to others around them, and unable to satisfy their needs through these relations, they are alienated from them all. (See especially K. Marx, *The Economic and Philosophic Manuscripts of 1844*, trans. M. Mulligan, [New York: International Publishers, 1964], pp138-141.)

page 90: For the purposes of this discussion, I shall refer most often to the organization of a typical department of internal medicine. Other departments do not differ significantly, except that they tend to be smaller.

page 91: Particularly in some American medical centres, this latter provision can prove very lucrative to the experienced physician who knows his or her worth.

page 93: A fourth heart sound is only occasionally of major diagnostic significance and is even more rarely of value in determining therapy. It is just one of those clinical findings that adds to the wisdom and credibility of sub-specialists and enhances their sense of authority. (See B.W. Cobbs Jr., "Clinical recognition and medical management of rheumatic heart disease and other acquired valvular disease", in J.W. Hurst, *The Heart*, third edition [New York: McGraw-Hill, 1974], p917.)

page 95: Ophthalmologists also love to play this game with their elderly cataract patients.

page 96: An allied phenomenon is the unwillingness of most resident staff to take very strong exception to something an attending physician says. Most faculty members let it be known to what extent they appreciate dissent and discussion and what behaviour is appropriate in their presence. Their wishes are usually respected. Such a compliant attitude on the part of house officers is not new. Before establishing his famous clinic in Minnesota at the beginning of this century, William Mayo visited many medical schools on the eastern seaboard. The status of the house officers in these institutions did not impress him: "They seem to spend their days in subservient yessir-ing, in being flunkies for the permanent staff." (See H. Clapesattle, *The Mayo Brothers* [Boston: Houghton Mifflin, 1962], p521.)

page 97: That same summer, a major medical journal came out with a report on the treatment of malignant insulinomas based on experience with 52 patients. (See L.E. Broder, S.K. Carter, "Pancreatic islet cell carcinoma, II: results of therapy with streptozotocin in 52 patients", *Annals of Internal Medicine* 79 [1973]: 108-118.)

page 100: Medical educators are well aware of the physician-in-training's need for aggrandizement. When they apply for internships, medical students may be told — as I was in a few places — that "this is an interns' hospital", meaning that the interns make the decisions about patient care. In spite of such assurances, this is hardly ever true, especially in university hospitals. The weight of opinion from above is so great that interns have little choice but to comply with the 'suggestions' of their superiors. This restriction on their independent activity inevitably makes it more difficult for house officers to learn their trade.

In some hospitals, though, particularly municipal hospitals, the interns *are* given considerable independence and responsibility, thus giving rise to the opposite problem: a good deal of their learning in this situation is at the expense of their patients.

page 102: Recently, some nurses have been given the opportunity to advance to a level intermediate between nurse and physician, called "nurse-practitioner". Their numbers are very few, however, and further upgrading is still not possible.

page 103: I will never forget one nurse I met on a rotation during which I spent some time "scrubbing" for the operating room. The woman who supervised the operating theatres was a dynamo I shall name Beefeater. Ms. Beefeater was an uncompromising autocrat, the absolute, unquestioned, omnipotent and omniscient authority in all instances. Medical students and interns who crossed her path learned very rapidly not to dare question her judgement about anything. She was particularly fussy about operating room attire. It is reported that she once denied access to the cardiac arrest team, who had come to attempt to revive a patient, because they were not dressed properly for the occasion. Whether the issue at hand was costume or conduct, however, Nurse Beefeater's word was absolute. Her judgement, which was based on considerable experience, was often quite sound. At other times, she exercised authority just for the sake of demonstrating the girth of her biceps. The senior residents were able to get along with her without having to humiliate themselves very often but it was only the chief of the department who could dominate her consistently.

page 104: Soon thereafter, medical students begin to assume responsibility by making decisions, often requiring that they give instructions (orders) to people with as much or more experience than themselves. Medical students thrive on this responsibility.

page 105: Not nearly so serious, but equally instructive, is a phenomenon common to the experience of all interns and residents. Typically, in the middle of the night, the house officer receives a telephone call from the nurse on a ward. "I am sorry to bother you, Doctor," she says, "but Mrs. Alzheimer has fallen out of bed again. Could you please come and examine her and fill out an accident report?" In my experience, this sort of request almost always came just after I had fallen asleep. In *The Year of the Intern*, one of Robin Cook's major complaints is being dragged out of bed repeatedly for such mundane work. Although it is evidently something Cook has thought about a great deal, he does not demonstrate very much understanding of the underlying causes of the problem. He admits that "the nurses know what to do," but then proceeds to blame the hospital authorities for what he considers to be silly rules about filling in reports in the middle of the night: "This sort of thing is simply hazing and harassment, a kind of initiation rite into the American Medical Association." (See R. Cook, *Year of the Intern* [New York: Harcourt, Brace, Jovanovitch, 1972; Signet edition, 1973], pp46-47.)

There is a certain amount of truth in what Cook says. The long hours worked do play a part in socializing student physicians into their future role, just as do many other aspects of their training, but to suggest that the ordeals they endure are part of a plot to torment and to indoctrinate future physicians is highly inaccurate. Interns who are awakened in the middle of the night to perform mundane tasks are merely experiencing one consequence of the allocation of authority in the hospital. This problem will be frequently encountered in any situation where the rights and responsibilities of people are defined in relation to a hierarchy.

5

Just What
The Doctor Ordered

rounds and Rounds and Patient Management

One spring while I was an undergraduate in medical school I attended the convocation ceremony for that particular year's graduating class. While the whole affair tended to be histrionic, as expected at that type of function, the most pretentious item on the programme was a speech by the class valedictorian.

"Today is a great day for all of us," said the young physician. "But there is an even greater one yet to come. It will be . . . late one night on the wards of the Massachusetts General, in the emergency room of the Vancouver General, in the outpatient department of the Royal Vic. That very important day will be the one on which we first make decisions on our own. That is what this training and this degree are all about."

"He's been watching a little too much Dr. Kildare," I thought at the time. Not until later did I realize how close to the mark that newly-annointed Doctor of Medicine was in assessing the degree to which many physicians cherish their unique, rarely challenged authority to make decisions concerning the lives and health of other people. In fact, this sense of authority has become so completely accepted by most people that it takes special effort to realize how little it is based on medical necessity, and how much on the distorted requirements of hospitals and the personal motivations of physicians themselves.

Authority in medical practice is not directed exclusively towards patients. As we have seen already, other targets may include most of those who share the physician's working life: nurses, students, orderlies and other health workers. At the same time physicians are obliged to submit themselves to other more senior of their own colleagues in the complex hospital hierarchy.

This chapter explores what this hierarchical top-heavy medical structure means in terms of everyday practice. As illustration, it looks at the ritual of hospital "rounds" and, secondly, at that most helpless victim of the physician's authority, the patient.

rounds and Rounds: rituals in hospital medical practice

Interpersonal relationships in the hospital are often far from healthy, as we have seen, but the responsibility for this does not rest exclusively with the people involved, because their interactions with others are rarely spontaneous and unstructured. The working day of physicians is in fact highly structured, and the quanta of preplanned activity that occupy so much of their time go by the name of **rounds.**

Hospital rounds are something special. So rigidly do they follow a prescribed formula, and so integral are they to hospital life — at least as far as physicians are concerned — that they are of interest for their ritualistic aspects at least as much as for the educational experience they ostensibly provide.

Two quite different types of rounds deserve attention: "rounds" (with a small "r") occurring on the wards of a hospital and associated with the day-to-day care of patients, and "Rounds", which are conferences principally held as teaching exercises.

rounds: working on the ward

Ward rounds differ considerably from one hospital to the next and particularly, from one specialty to another. On a given ward, they might be conducted in any of a number of different ways depending on the time of day, the presence or absence of a staff or attending physician and the inclinations of the participants. The most frequent format for rounds is that of the so-called work rounds, which are co-ordinated by the senior resident on the ward and at which the attending physician is not present. These rounds are generally held every morning and, on some wards, every evening as well.

On general medical (that is, internal medicine) wards, rounds can easily last all morning. They begin first thing after the house staff has drawn blood specimens and rewritten expired prescription orders.*

On most wards, the patients' records are filed in a chart-rack on wheels; the signal to commence is the rolling of this rack to one end of the corridor by the chief resident. The house staff then gather around in loose formation and rounds are under way.

The intern who has been caring for the patient in the first bed begins (out of the patient's hearing): "Mrs. Dumont is a forty-nine year old French Canadian lady who was admitted to the hospital nine days ago with an acute myocardial infarction [a heart attack]. She developed congestive heart failure, but has been well controlled with digoxin and diuretics."

The senior resident then may ask a few questions about the patient's progress. What are her enzyme levels today (looking for evidence of ongoing damage to the heart)? When was her last electrocardiogram and what did it show? What is her stage of mobilization? All of these questions are very practical. In more academic centres, the discussion will frequently move from the particular to the universal and, often, to the relatively esoteric: Have you read the recent article in the New England Journal on the ear-lobe sign in coronary artery disease? Did you see the editorial published in The Lancet last week which weighed the current evidence on the role for hormones in the development of atherosclerosis?"

Rules of conduct are rigorously observed during rounds and senior residents play a key role in establishing mood. If a particular senior resident wants the rounds to be brisk and matter-of-fact, they are; if a resident wants them to be leisurely and academic, they are. It is the resident who signals the move from one room to the next by pushing the chart-rack along the corridor. Other house officers may occasionally push it but only when there is no doubt that a move is about to be made. The senior resident frequently leans over the chart-rack while the cases are being discussed. The other house officers usually stand erect or lean against the corridor walls.

The amount of time devoted to the more academic matters very much depends on what else is happening. If new patients are being admitted or if there is someone on the ward who is very sick, rounds are conducted much more quickly. Most participants in rounds are conscious of the need to order the necessary investigations and to institute the proper therapy, but beyond that, their major concern is that their work (and the rounds) be as interesting as possible.

That, of course, is reasonable and understandable but it does have consequences for patient care. Rounds that are entirely oriented to the practical are rarely very interesting, and they must last longer if the "interesting stuff" is to be touched upon. This means, among other things, time that might have been spent with patients — getting to know them as people and discussing their problems with them — is devoted instead to the pursuit of intellectual interests. This does not necessarily mean that the adequacy of patient care suffers, because one consequence of extensive rounds is that the negligence of a house officer cannot easily be overlooked.* On the other hand, the commonly voiced complaint of patients that they have minimal contact with their physicians in hospital and the fact that house officers often do not get around to explaining to many of their patients what is going on, both bear some relationship to the amount of time taken up by long periods spent on rounds.

Senior residents also decide the priority to be accorded each patient: whether to linger or to pass by quickly, whether to confer in the corridor or go to the bedside and examine the patient. A number of factors enter into this decision: the complexity of a case and any controversy surrounding treatment; the seriousness of a patient's condition; and the interest which a particular case holds for the resident.

Another consequence of "academic" rounds is that physicians may talk themselves into unnecessary investigations of some patients just to satisfy their own curiosity. Occasionally, this leads to invasive and dangerous procedures (for example, a case I encountered of a woman with a fever who underwent heart catheterization because one physician was impressed by the prominence of the veins in her neck). Much more often, in my experience, a hospital stay is prolonged to allow the accumulation of data unlikely to be of any benefit to the patient. Often as well the "interesting" patient is allowed to stay longer in the hospital, recuperating, than a person with a run-of-the-mill problem. Residents work in the hospital for much less money than they could earn as general practitioners: the opportunity to learn is their major justification for being there. They know that the interesting cases, from which they learn the most, are important for the specialty certification examinations.

The perspective underlying such interactions with patients is one which treats them as impersonal objects of care and, even more so, of educational experience. The format of rounds encourages the development of such an attitude, to the point where I have heard residents say on more than one occasion: "Let's get that patient out of here; we aren't learning anything from him anymore."

Senior residents usually jot down the major decisions taken during rounds and the important tasks to be done afterwards. A nurse along on rounds may take notes on matters relevant to nursing care. This is about all a nurse who braves rounds ever gets to do, although once in a while a question about a particular patient might be directed towards her. Nurses are not encouraged to participate in rounds, which are strictly the affair of physicians and physicians-in-training. Typically, a nurse who shows up at the beginning of rounds will wander off after an hour or two of pained silence.

As for other hospital workers, it would be unthinkable for them to be present on rounds. Even though an orderly or nursing assistant might know a patient best and have some important insight about how a patient is doing or would feel about a proposed procedure, most physicians would not know how to begin to ask such workers for their opinions.

Even less permissible is the involvement of patients in discussions about their own cases. Either a closed door stands between them and discussion or else the physicians mumble discreetly out of earshot — in spite of the fact that these deliberations might decide the patient's fate. Some rather important decisions are made during rounds: a patient should or should not have a particular procedure; a patient should or should not be allowed to die. The house officers decide such matters in consultation with the attending physician, while patients are rarely aware of the therapeutic options available.

Not only are patients denied the opportunity to participate in discussions vital to their well-being; rounds are structured in a way that minimizes the opportunity for *any* kind of interaction between physician and patient. The physicians, mulling over the problems outside the patients' rooms, usually succeed in abstracting themselves from a patient's particular reality. If they have any doubts about the 'clinical signs' or symptoms, they may go into the room and ask a pertinent question or two, take pokes in turn at the patient's belly or listen to the heart; that done, they leave the room to continue their deliberations. If there is no special reason to examine or interview a patient on a particular day, that patient may be graced with no more than a perfunctory nod or a few words on the latest decisions about what lies ahead.

The ritual of rounds depersonalizes care. Medical care has come a long way from the days when any decisions about therapy were made by the physician, at the bedside, holding the patient's hand with the family gathered around. Decisions have become more complex, of course, but it is not necessary to take the decisions concerning care further away from the patient because of this. When a decision is made in a corridor, out of earshot, among a group of physicians who do not really know the patient, the likelihood of a sensitive and humane decision is inevitably diminished.*

The callousness and indifference of many house officers towards their patients is fostered by their attending physicians. One time, when riding in a hospital elevator, I overheard two senior physicians discussing the ward with which they were both affiliated.

"Lots of interesting cases these days," said one, the head of a subspecialty division.

"Yes, we have excellent teaching material on the ward," replied the Chief of Service, referring, of course, to the *people* under his care. The face of one visitor to the hospital who was riding in that elevator revealed his surprise at the conversation, but it was something not many house officers would have found unusual. In fact, when viewed from the depersonalized perspective of ward rounds, patients become little more than teaching material. And ward rounds are frequently the only time patients are seen by physicians during the course of a day.

Sometimes during rounds a doctor will make an inadvertent remark that reveals to a patient for the first time a certain aspect of his or her condition or therapy — without the physician realizing this has happened. Once an intern I was working with made a comment to the attending physician as we were leaving a patient's bedside: "The tumour is involving his pancreas." They nodded to each other knowingly and left the room; neither looked towards the patient, who had previously been unaware of his grave condition: his heart was sinking through the floor.

On another occasion a surgical resident remarked to his attending physician that the patient whose bed they were walking past was scheduled for surgery the next day. This was the first the patient had heard of the operation, but no one stopped to explain to him what was going on (until later in the day when, presumably, an intern or resident had to come around to obtain signed 'consent' for the procedure).

The ritual of going through all the rooms on the ward, and of at least nodding in the direction of each patient helps physicians convince themselves that they are devoting enough time and attention to each patient even when this is not the case. This is, to use Ivan Illich's formulation, a sort of ritualization of progress.*

The attending physicians who evaluate the performance of house officers do not often look beyond what happens on rounds to assess the quality of the care they have been delivering: those who can perform well on rounds are home free. William Nolen gives a good illustration of this in *The Making of a Surgeon:*

[Rounds were] the intern's chance to shine, his opportunity to score the points he needed for reappointment, and neither I nor anyone else interfered unless he was obviously passing out a large pile of misinformation.

We had one intern who would occasionally do this. If he didn't know the answer he'd make it up. He was a smooth operator, and he got away with it for quite a while...[1]

Nolen goes on to describe how this intern would bluff his way through laboratory values he couldn't remember. But one day he got caught describing a physical finding that did not exist. The rules of rounds on Nolen's service were that no one would interfere with such performances by a young physician, who might well have been negligent at a patient's expense. It is for the benefit of physicians that rounds are held, and patients are not always their highest priority.

Surgeons prefer that their house officers are able to rattle off laboratory values during rounds. Doctors in internal medicine place less emphasis on these and look instead upon outside readings as the measure of competence. One article quoted from the *British Heart Journal* is worth any number of cardiac enzyme levels committed to memory.

Surgical rounds are different in another way: they begin much earlier and end much sooner. When I worked on surgical wards, where rounds began at seven instead of eight or even nine on a medical ward, I found that if I arrived at five after seven I would have missed half of rounds. Surgeons whiz through rounds with nary a word to their patients: just examine the wound, feel the belly, check the fluid intake and the temperature chart, draw the bloods, and order the medications, in this way disposing of the whole ward in half an hour; then it's down to the cafeteria for some breakfast before the first case in the operating room. If the resident does not have any operations scheduled that day rounds do not become more leisurely, but breakfast often does.

Rounds: le spectacle

If ward rounds terminate at noon, it is usually because the house officers are on their way to Rounds, or those conferences that go on primarily as a function of teaching. Depending on the day of the week, the house officers might be off to a conference for the physicians affiliated with their ward (Service Rounds); a conference dealing with a particular subspecialty (Cardiology Rounds, Immunology Rounds); or the major weekly conference in their specialty (Medical Grand Rounds, Surgical Grand Rounds). Principally intended to inform and teach, on the average day there are two or more such conferences in a department of internal medicine alone. Of course, not all the house officers are present at each conference. But it is usual for them each to attend at least one of these hour-long Rounds nearly every day.

The senior resident on any ward or subspecialty service handles the organization of Rounds in his department. Grand Rounds are planned by the chief resident in the specialty (although some surgical services do not allow their chief residents this much responsibility!).

In those hospitals where Rounds are a big thing — generally, the academic hospitals — the resident responsible spends a great deal of time planning and organizing the conference. The preparation consists of selecting a case or cases for discussion, informing medical students or interns who have been involved in the care of patients that they must present a case, informing one or more faculty members about the topic for Rounds and asking them to be prepared to discuss some aspect of it, acquiring any equipment needed for audiovisual presentations and, occasionally, reserving a room. That is a lot of work for any one person, particularly one who has many other responsibilities, so it is not uncommon for the resident to begin planning one week's conference the day after the previous one, or even sooner.

The role of medical students or interns is to distil all the pertinent data into a concise presentation. In some hospitals, house officers are expected to present cases without referring to notes and have to memorize the presentation. Frequently, they must prepare slides to accompany the talk. All in all, everyone involved in a particular Rounds spends many hours preparing for the occasion. The time spent is usually proportional to the importance of the Rounds, Grand Rounds requiring the most preparation of all.

In the conference room, the first row of seats is the preserve of the senior physicians. Occasionally the senior resident, whose active role in the Rounds is now over, will breach this rank. Behind these people sit the rank and file of junior attending physicians and house officers in the division. The rest of the seats are occupied by an assortment of attending physicians and house officers who are not part of the immediate hierarchy of the division holding the conference, but are attending out of interest.

The chief of the service, division or department (in the case of Medical Grand Rounds, this is the physician-in-chief) introduces the topic under discussion and each person who is to speak. The Rounds begins with a case presentation, the Moment of Glory for the student or intern. There is a very particular format for these presentations. One of my colleagues once commented that he felt like a schoolboy every time he stood there in his white uniform, reciting a case in the preordained way:

A sixty-three year old man came to the hospital complaining of shortness of breath of three hours duration...

He was perfectly well prior to the onset of the episode that precipitated admission. There was no previous history of...

On examination, he was an alert, well developed man, looking his age, slightly cyanotic [blue], *in mild respiratory distress. His respiratory rate was...*

Laboratory investigations showed a white count of 9900, with a normal differential count; blood enzymes were normal; there was a marked depression in the C_3 and total hemolytic complement . . .

The patient was managed conservatively [he received no therapy], *and improved steadily. Respiratory symptoms disappeared on the fifth hospital day, and he was discharged four days later with a final diagnosis of . . ."*

This format is followed rigorously: chief complaint, history of present illness, functional inquiry, laboratory data, course in hospital, discharge diagnosis. House officers do not comment upon the case. Using this format, they are able to convey the clinical data quite efficiently.

Obviously, certain things will rarely, if ever, enter into such a presentation: the social and psychological background to a patient's disease; the effect of the illness on the patient and family and work relationships; socio-economic factors making it unlikely that the patient will comply with certain therapy; and so on. These are not the matters that have brought specialists and students to the conference room; the doctors and students are there to be 'stimulated intellectually', but only in a very narrow sense.

The room is usually darkened during the house officer's presentation so slides can be projected. Generally the slides echo the presentation word for word. I have never understood why this is done; it is as though the audience was incapable of following an oral presentation, perhaps, or could not trust a house officer unless the slides were there to lend authority to the words.

The room is darkened once again when the radiologist takes to the podium to present x-rays. Then come one or more other specialists who also play to a darkened chamber and use slides to back themselves up.

This constant flashing of slides and dimming of lights contributes to the authoritarian nature of Rounds: the authority of the presenter and the passivity of the audience are maximized. The visual material confronts the audience as a *fait accompli*, a statement of what is important in relation to the case under discussion. That is not to say that members of the audience will not express disagreement with points raised; frequently they do. What happens almost invariably, though, is that the spectators accept the terms of discussion established by the speakers.

It is quite consistent with the prominent role of authority in Rounds that the opinion of a member of the audience is respected in proportion to rank, that the final word on any controversial subject is sought by the physician-in-chief from the head of the appropriate subspecialty division, and that no one oversteps the bounds of authority in expounding a view or in criticising a colleague.

Of course, most physicians are quite happy with the orientation and priorities, as well as with the aesthetics and organization of Rounds. Similarly, most physicians are content with the emphasis of most conferences on the 'interesting case', which means that diseases like Waldenstrom's macroglobulinemia and polyarteritis nodosa are heard from at least as often as commonplace diseases like chronic bronchitis and cirrhosis of the liver. Not all conferences deal with esoterica, but even when Rounds focuses on a common disorder, disproportionate attention is paid to its more 'interesting' aspects — rare complications and the like. Only the occasional Rounds is genuinely and entirely oriented to the practical.

Some of the more 'liberal' department or division heads encourage the occasional conference on a 'relevant' subject so as to make up for the lack of attention given to it otherwise. A friend of mine related a rather amusing encounter he had with the chief of his clinical department while he was interning. One day he was summoned to the chief's office (certainly not something that happened very often).

The chief came right to the point. "John, I've been thinking that we really ought to find out what is going on in those community clinics," he began. "I understand you've been working in association with the one in Pointe Ste. Charles."

"Yes, that's right," the intern replied.

"Well, why don't we have a Rounds on the clinic. You could make a presentation on it, couldn't you?"

"I think that if you want to hear about the clinic, it should be from the citizens and health workers who work there," John said.

"I see," replied the Professor finishing the discussion and never opening it again. Nor was such a Rounds ever held in that hospital.

My friend had two observations on this encounter. The first was that handing over a conference to the control of outsiders is alien to the medical mind. That is, any subject to be discussed must be treated in the familiar way. His second conclusion was that the chief thought it possible to do justice to a much neglected subject by holding one Rounds on it. It is through such carefully controlled exposure in the traditional ritual format of Rounds that physicians may succeed in convincing themselves that they are paying adequate attention to a problem they otherwise ignore.*

The extent to which all but strictly academic considerations are excluded from the conference room was underlined for me on one occasion during my internship. On a Wednesday, I was scheduled to present a case at Medical Grand Rounds. On the Tuesday before, a military junta overthrew the democratically-elected government of Chile, killing the president of the country and, ultimately, thousands of others. I had been interested in the socialist experiment in Chile, even planning to go to work there after my internship. Naturally, these events upset me considerably.

When I arose at Rounds the next day, I began: "I cannot make my presentation without first taking a moment to pay respect to the memory of Salvador Allende, the late President of Chile, who did so much to uphold the spirit of Hippocrates [Allende was a physician]."

I then went on with my presentation, a case of carbamazepine-induced inappropriate antidiuresis, thinking that no one would take offence at my remarks. But afterwards a number of my colleagues asked me how I had the nerve to say such a thing at Rounds. One (exaggerating somewhat, I hope) commented that some attending physicians sitting near him had clenched their teeth and had visibly perspired while I spoke. Several months later, an intern who had not been there that day asked me if it were true that I had really said what had been reputed. And, *over a year after the Rounds*, I was introduced to one of the attending physicians outside of the hospital; on hearing my name, he asked: "Aren't you the one who was always talking about Chile?"

In retrospect, I realize that I should not have made that statement at Rounds: it was hardly the place to begin a political crusade, and I certainly wasn't going to win over any converts. Political commentary is alien to Rounds, but that is not to say that Rounds do not have politcal overtones. Rounds are allegedly unideological, but they are not. Their ideology is an unquestioning acceptance of the social, political and economic status quo. Rounds school physicians in the avoidance of broader social concerns and teach them an approach to medicine that ignores its socio-political context.

The ritual nature, rigid format and narrow focus of Rounds does more than just orient the physician in this way. Rounds are authoritarian and encourage passivity amongst those in attendance. It is instructive to consider the similarities between Rounds and other authoritarian spectacles:

[Fascist aesthetics] flow from [and justify] a preoccupation with situations of control, submissive behaviour, and extravagant effort; they exalt two seemingly opposite states, egomania and servitude. The relations of domination and enslavement take the form of characteristic pageantry: the massing of groups of people; the turning of people into things; the multiplication of things and grouping of people/things around an all-powerful, hypnotic leader figure or force. The fascist dramaturgy centers on the orgiastic transactions between mighty forces and their puppets. Its choreography alternates between ceaseless motion and congealed, static 'virile' posing. Fascist art glorifies surrender; it exalts mindlessness; it glamorizes death.

Such art is hardly confined to works labelled as fascist or produced under fascist governments . . .[2]

It would be ludicrous to suggest that the spectacle of Rounds is as orgiastic or enslaving as Hitler's Nuremberg Rally (which is being described in part of the above text), but there are certain parallels: the staging and 'choreography' of the event, the lulling of the audience into submission before the authority of the leader. Of course, Rounds are *not* a plot to capture the minds of physicians. Nevertheless, just as the rituals of fascism fulfilled a need (often, the need to submit) in the citizens who attended, so does the ritual of Rounds fulfil, in some way, the needs of physicians.

One further observation must be made about Rounds: like *rounds*, they are the preserve of physicians and medical students. Other health workers rarely venture into these conferences, and when they do they undoubtedly find it very difficult to follow the discussion, because presentations are not aimed at their level. This exclusivity is quite consistent with the lack of priority given by physicians to the sharing of knowledge and the discussing of cases with other health workers. Indeed, this unshared body of knowledge is the source of much of the physician's power.

Patient management

Mrs. Goldblatt* is a forty-six year old woman who came over to a booth we had set up in a shopping centre to check blood pressures. Her reading was 180 millimetres over 110 millimetres, a significant elevation. Normal blood pressure is less than 140 over 90. A person with hypertension – a persistently elevated blood pressure – has, if untreated, a much greater risk than normal of strokes and other serious diseases.

I asked Mrs. Goldblatt if she had ever had an elevated blood pressure reading before.

"Oh, the doctor never tells me what my blood pressure is," she replied. "Whenever he checks it, he says it's a little high, but that it's all right for me to have high blood pressure because I'm nervous."

"Did your physician ever do any tests on you to see why your blood pressure was elevated?"

"No."

"Did he tell you to come back at regular intervals so he could check it?"

"No."

"*Did he have you lie down or relax for ten or fifteen minutes on any occasion before checking your blood pressure?*"

"*I don't think he's ever spent ten minutes with me.*"

"Well," I said less hopefully, "*I guess he hasn't taught you or anyone in your family how to measure blood pressure, so it could be checked at home when you would be less nervous.*"

"*Me? Measure blood pressure? Do you think he should have?*"

I explained the consequences of untreated hypertension to Mrs. Goldblatt. She agreed to go to the hospital clinic for a repeat examination and, possibly, to be started on therapy.

Roughly speaking, doctors make decisions about patient care or therapy in three stages. First, they have to decide if the patient is in fact ill. Second, if a disease is diagnosed, doctors must decide if therapy is warranted. Finally, if there is to be a "therapeutic intervention", doctors decide on the specific form this intervention will take.

In Mrs. Goldblatt's case the physician, on his own, made a "first-stage" decision. He used his "clinical judgement" to decide that her elevated readings were a manifestation of nervousness and not of the disease, hypertension. He did not attempt to develop a strategy with his patient to discover what her blood pressure readings were when she was less nervous than he presumed her to be at the time of his examination. Nor did he inform her of the potential seriousness of untreated hypertension. Had he done so, she might have pressed him to arrive at a diagnosis based more on observation than on intuition. In this case, the intuition of the physician was probably incorrect.*

Mr. Atherton is a sixty-year-old man I saw in a surgery clinic. Three months before this visit he had undergone what was then quite a new operation: a vein from his leg was transplanted to his chest, where it was put into place as an artery to increase the supply of blood to the heart. This operation is sometimes performed on people who have angina — incapacitating chest pain — associated with exertion; in the majority of cases, the operation relieves the pain. At the time Mr. Atherton was operated on, as a result of the surgery there was a one-in-twenty risk of death in the month after the operation. Because of this, and because the operation had not proven to prolong lives of patients even though relieving their symptoms, the procedure remained controversial.

Mr. Atherton came into the examining room with his wife. I asked him how he was doing.

"Much better," he replied. *"I've had no pain since the operation. It's hard to believe."*

After I had examined him and expressed my satisfaction with his progress, he looked at his wife, then back at me, and said: "Doc, there's something I've been meaning to ask. What's the difference between arteries and veins? If they took a vein out of my leg, how do I get the blood that I need down there?"

I suspect that my expression betrayed astonishment. At that early stage of my career (I was in the third year of my medical studies) I assumed that the patient would have been given a detailed explanation beforehand of precisely what so important and dangerous an operation involved. He would have been told how it was supposed to help him, as well as the indications and contra-indications for surgery and the alternatives to it. Or so I thought.

"Didn't someone discuss this with you before the operation?" I asked.

"No."

I explained that blood leaves the heart through the arteries and returns through the veins, and that the veins are less crucial. There are so many veins that the blood can find an alternate route if one is missing.

"Then why did they put a vein in my heart if veins are not really very important?"

I told him that the vein had been connected to the aorta, the main artery, and to the coronary artery on the heart, and that the vein was, therefore, functioning as an artery, bringing more blood to the heart muscle and increasing its ability to tolerate exercise without precipitating angina.

"Surely someone explained all this to you before?" I asked him.

"No. They only told me that I had to have this operation, that they would take a vein from my leg and put it in my heart. They said there was some risk with the operation but that I had to have it if I was to go back to work."

Mr. Atherton's surgery was the result of a 'second-stage' decision; that is, a decision that the patient is ill and therapy is warranted. The decision was made without consulting him and without any suggestion that alternative courses might exist. In fact, although the diagnosis was clear-cut in his case, the decision to operate was not. He was not told about the probable benefits of the operation (relief of symptoms but not necessarily an increase in life expectancy) or of possible drawbacks (the five per cent risk of death). If all of these things had been explained to him, he would have been in a better position to make his own decisions, to determine if he wanted to take his chances with the surgery or, perhaps, seek the opinion of another physician.*

Mrs. Cooper, fifty-one years old, was admitted to hospital after notic-
ing a lump in her left breast. She was examined by a surgeon, a resident and
a student, and they all believed that the lump, hard and irregular as it was,
was probably malignant. In spite of this, the woman was informed that the
lump was most likely benign, and that "only in the remote possibility" that
it was found to be malignant at the time of biopsy would the doctors under-
take a more extensive operation, involving amputation of the breast.

The biopsy specimen was examined while the patient was still under
anaesthetic. As predicted, it was malignant and the surgeon proceded to
perform a modified radical mastectomy. This form of surgery involves re-
moval not only of the breast, but also of the nearby lymph glands. In
severity it is intermediate between a simple mastectomy (when only the breast
is removed) and a radical mastectomy (when the muscles underlying the breast
are removed along with the lymph glands and the breast itself.)

A common side effect of lymph gland removal is swelling of the
arm on the affected side. When muscles are removed as well, some
weakness of the arm is also incurred.

These three operations (simple, modified radical and radical
mastectomies) are in competition, in the sense that there are no
grounds at present for preferring any particular one unequivocally
over the others. Physicians who believe that available evidence does
not justify performing the more radical procedures, because of the
discomfort and inconvenience they entail, advocate the less extensive variants.

Notwithstanding this controversy, Mrs. Cooper was never advised that there were a number of possibilities, much less asked
which one she preferred.

In this case both the diagnosis and the necessity for therapy
were unarguable, but the 'stage-three' decision — which therapy to
employ — was not. To the surgeon the choice of operation may have
seemed academic, almost a matter of taste, especially in the absence
of reliable statistics on whether the more radical procedures significantly improve the prognosis. But the patient might have been
willing to tolerate a more extensive procedure for any possible additional benefit, however unproved. Or she may equally have chosen
to minimize the trauma of amputation by opting for the least drastic
of the three variants. But by telling her only that the possibility of
the major operation was remote, her physicians avoided involving
her in the decision at all.

Mrs. Pickwick, fifty-four years old, was admitted to the hospital be-
cause of uncontrolled diabetes. She was very obese, a condition the physi-

cians apparently felt was largely responsible for the lack of control of the diabetes. Overweight people often have problems handling the carbohydrates they consume unless they strictly follow a low-calorie diet.

Mrs. Pickwick had never followed her diet. And it was evident at the time of her admission that her blood sugar, consistently two or three times the normal value, could not be significantly reduced by the pills she had been taking, even though she was on the maximum dose.

These pills make a person's utilization of the insulin they produce more efficient. When they fail, the only alternative is to supplement the body's production of insulin with a supply of the hormone in injectable form. Obviously, this was going to be necessary if Mrs. Pickwick's blood sugar was to be normalized, but the resident in charge of her case was very apprehensive about doing so.

"I won't give it to her," he told us. "She is too stupid to take insulin. She has been so unco-operative with her treatment in the past that giving it to her would only make matters worse."

For two weeks the resident doctor made a gallant effort to control her blood sugar without giving her the hormone. To no one's surprise, it didn't work. Finally my colleague was forced to admit that, "Morally, we can't send this woman back into the street with a blood sugar way over two hundred. She refuses to follow a diet and the only way we can get her controlled is with insulin."

He discussed the case with several other physicians and a decision was taken to place her on insulin. The patient was never party to these discussions. After fifteen days in hospital, she was informed of the physicians' decisions. She was not asked at any time how she felt about taking insulin. Presumably, if the doctors had decided against giving it to her, she would never have known that it was even a possibility.

In Mrs. Pickwick's case, a series of 'stage-three' decisions was made by the physicians, based on their assessment of the likelihood of her compliance with each possible therapy. Had she been consulted, she might have indicated which form of therapy she would have been most willing and able to take. Indeed, if she had been involved in making decisions about therapy, and if the rationale for therapy had been properly explained to her, the likelihood of her compliance might have increased.

In each of the four cases described, the physician was able to deny the patient any significant role in an important diagnostic or therapeutic decision. This denial is characteristic of the way authority operates in the physician-patient relationship. It is widely regarded as a normal and even necessary part of that relationship, usually on the grounds that sound medical decisions can only be made by those with prolonged and intensive training.

But although physicians' specialized training may certainly make them valuable advisors, the necessity for this kind of relationship is not supported by the evidence. In fact, we do not have to look far to find reasons for encouraging increased involvement of patients in therapeutic decisions.

In the case of Mrs. Pickwick we have already encountered one compelling medical justification for involving the patient: the problem of controlling her diabetic condition could have been greatly simplified if she had been consulted about the choice of treatment; this simple consultation would have brought obvious benefits for herself as well as her physicians. Several studies in recent years indicate that patient compliance is regularly improved when doctors are willing to provide information concerning the disease and its treatment.[3] Keeping patients informed can sometimes even eliminate the need for treatment altogether.*

Another kind of consideration, though non-medical, should carry equal weight: the secondary effects of therapy on patients. Medical therapy can be a severe imposition upon the ways of life, self-images and psyches of persons who undergo it, often far more than physicians are aware. If lives are to be compromised, changed or even terminated by particular therapeutic choices, then it is surely the right of all persons to make their own decisions, to be provided with all the facts and to be made aware of the alternative courses of action.

In his *Profession of Medicine,* Harvard University sociologist Eliot Friedson provides a forceful expression of this point:

[It] is a social rather than a medical question to ask what degree of the convenience of the treated should be subordinated to the convenience of the treater, whether or not the treated should be provided with full information about alternative modes of management and treatment and the freedom to choose his mode, whether or not institutionalization should take place, and what the routines of management in institutions should be. For such issues, the profession is a rather special source of advice in that it is expert in what treatment is necessary and therefore what technical limits are imposed on the alternatives for management. But within these limits given, the alternatives remain a matter in which lay choice is quite legitimate and professional autonomy illegitimate.[4]

Friedson blames the tendency of physicians to make therapeutic decisions autonomously on the nature of professionalism:

When an occupation arises to serve some need on the part of the lay community and subsequently succeeds in becoming a profession, it gains the autonomy to become, at least in part, selfsustaining, equipped to turn back and shape, even create that need anew, defining, selecting and organizing the way it is expressed in social life.[5]

It is true, as Friedson says, that the unique status of the physicians gives them the opportunity to "control the terms and content of (their) work" and hence to dominate their patients. However, it remains to be explained why doctors trouble themselves to take advantage of this opportunity.

Quite early in the course of their training, medical students observe many examples of doctor-patient interaction, most of them dominated by the doctors. Beginning with their first experience at dissecting cadavers, they are taught to view patients as passive recipients of their professional activity. Then, in some phases of training, students are called upon to make decisions autonomously in emergency situations, often late at night with a patient too ill to participate in therapeutic decisions even if the opportunity were provided. The students learn that physicians save patients' lives, that they cure patients' diseases. They discover that even when patients die, it is because physicians have "lost" them.*

Students are taught how to 'take a patient's history' in a way that efficiently elicits the most useful information, and how to conduct a formal and systematic physical examination. After thus 'working up' a patient, students learn to synthesize the data into a differential diagnosis, and plan, on that basis, the investigations (laboratory tests, x-rays) and therapy. Plans for therapy are discussed in great detail with physicians and with other trainees, but patients are rarely consulted unless written permission is required for some procedure (such as an operation).*

Whatever their predispositions and presumptions, medical students find few models or mechanisms at their disposal for involving patients in decisions. Unlike history-taking and physical examinations, the skill of enhancing patient participation is not taught in any organized way. And medical students newly arrived on hospital wards do not see very many people about them actively involving patients in their own care. It is little wonder that years of exposure to this situation lead students to regard treatment as a physician-centred process.

Physicians may rationalize their failures to discuss with patients the therapeutic options or their own uncertainties about diagnosis and treatment with that most humane of explanations: burdening patients in this way merely creates anxiety. That this is not the real explanation for physicians' reticence is evidenced by the fact that not all patients are treated the same.

Factors that influence the likelihood of physicians bringing patients in on their decisions include the physicians' own assessments of a particular patient's intelligence, awareness, emotional stability and apparent interest in the treatment of his or her disorder. And a doctor's assessment of all these factors bears some relationship to the patient's social class background.* In general, people from middle-class or upper-class backgrounds tend to articulate better what they want to know from doctors. People from the lower socio-economic groups are more likely to attempt to communicate their needs and wishes non-verbally — in their tone of voice, their facial expression or by what they leave unsaid.[6] Because physicians usually come from backgrounds themselves where non-verbal communication is less developed, they have trouble understanding the needs of people who do communicate in this way. And the recognition and interpretation of non-verbal communication is not, needless to say, a skill taught in medical school. I recall countless times when I related more openly to a patient whom I considered to be intelligent, articulate and interesting, or perhaps who asked me for specific information, than I did to one whom I sensed would be less able to grasp what I was talking about, or was simply less interested in doing so.

The idea of physician dominance receives another kind of reinforcement when students of medicine encounter the prevailing attitudes among colleagues towards patients who are women. It has been well documented that women are frequently portrayed in stereotypical and unflattering ways in medical lectures:

Following the traditional linguistic convention, patients in most medical school lectures are referred to exclusively by the male pronoun, 'he'. There is, however, a notable exception: in discussing a hypothetical patient whose disease is of psychogenic origin, the lecturer often automatically uses 'she'. For it is widely taught, both explicitly and implicitly, that women patients (when they receive notice at all) have uninteresting illnesses, are unreliable historians, and are beset by such emotionality that their symptoms are unlikely to reflect 'real' disease.[7]

The training received by the students or house officers, combined with any preexisting sexual prejudice, often results in lower standards of health care for women than for men. Mary Howell of Harvard University reports that:

1) Women, as compared to men, are more likely to have their depressions and anxieties treated by drugs than to be helped to overcome the cause of their distress. Indeed... symptoms of physical illness reported by women are often assumed to be of psychologic origin, and so treated.

2) The first cause of death for middle-aged adults of both sexes is cardiovascular disease. The not-too-distant second cause for women is breast carcinoma; respiratory disease is the less common second cause for men. Most conscientious physicians listen to the heart and lungs of every patient they examine, whatever the presenting complaint; relatively few so

routinely examine breasts and teach breast self-examination, although the latter is probably the most efficacious low-cost preventive (case-finding) measure for any of the three major causes of death.

3) In a study of patients in a hospital where "a complete examination was mandated by the hospital's medical board as well as by the State Department of Health," the most frequently omitted part of the admission physical was the pelvic examination.[8]

Ellen Frankfurt, an American journalist who has worked for the *Village Voice*, suggests that even women who are 'favoured' with pelvic examinations are treated in a degrading and depersonalizing way, for which there is no parallel in the medical care received by men:

The only way a man can understand the feelings a woman has towards a gynecologist is to put himself in her place. As a young adolescent he visits a doctor: all the people who answer the phone, make appointments, fill in charts and file them are male; only the person who sees him naked and examines him is female. During the examination he must lie on his back with his feet in the air while she inserts a cold instrument and then two fingers inside him. Throughout she is silent. When the examination is over she speaks: "You may get dressed now." Before leaving, the young man makes his appointment with the male receptionist.[9]

In the gynecology outpatient clinic where I learned to perform pelvic examinations, the set-up was about as depersonalized as one could imagine, and the outrage and indignation of at least some women were evident. After a brief interview by a resident physician or a medical student in a common room, where her 'history' could be overheard by other physicians, students and patients, each woman was shown into an examining 'room', which consisted of a bed, separated from others like it only by curtains. The conduct of the examination was very much as Frankfurt describes it, with an added feature: because the clinic was in a 'teaching hospital', the woman in stirrups had no way of knowing how many pairs of fingers would be inserted before she was allowed to get dressed.

In this kind of situation patients, male and female alike, are able to participate in health care only in the most passive sense while students and physicians come to regard them as nothing more than the object of their professional activity.* But, as the saying goes, it takes two to tango. Even though physicians may seek to dominate their patients, why must patients necessarily co-operate by submitting? Well, not all do.

Mrs. Romanoff is a woman of sixty-four who came to the hospital clinic, where she was seen by an intern. When the intern came into the room where she was waiting, Mrs. Romanoff spoke up before he could say a word.

"I came to see you because I am coughing," she said. "I want a chest x-ray. I don't want a lecture from you about my weight. If you give me any bullshit I'll leave."

Clearly, not all patients will submit to the physician's authority, and some will resist it vigorously. Often, however, it is difficult to resist. In situations where access to other doctors is difficult, the decision to seek alternative care cannot be taken lightly. Many patients are left in the frustrating position of being unable to get as much information or to participate as fully in care as they would like.

On the other hand, some patients are only too willing to bow down before the man with the mantle of Hippocrates.

Mr. Curley is a seventy year old widower who was admitted to the hospital for the third time in six weeks because of congestive heart failure. When he arrived the nurse on duty, who knew him well, confided to the intern that he was probably up to his old trick of not taking his medication so he could get into hospital. Subsequent blood tests bore out her prediction. Mr. Curley recovered rapidly with appropriate treatment, but whenever the possibility of leaving the hospital was raised, he became very anxious and claimed to be having a recurrence of his symptoms. When questioned about this, he admitted that he enjoyed the attention he received in the hospital and the sense of security he got from being there.

Like Mr. Curley, many patients are anxious to submit to the authority of the physician, or at least are willing to accept it. Talcott Parsons, author of *The Social System*, suggests that these people adopt a "sick role" as a form of permissible deviance from acceptable conduct in society. This role, regulated and legitimated by physicians, relieves the person who adopts it of many fundamental social obligations.[10]

H.B. Waitzkin and B. Waterman, in their study, *The Exploitation of Illness in Capitalist Society*, emphasize the stabilizing influence that the sick role can have on a social order, by allowing discontent to be diffused and defused through legitimate channels. In prisons and in totalitarian societies, for example, access to the sick role allows people to deviate without disrupting the world around them. Their sense of oppression is thereby lessened without leading to open expressions of discontent.[11]

Sick role behaviour also occurs in the everyday world of job-holding. Absenteeism due to illness is a commonly accepted measure of the dissatisfaction of workers with their jobs; management nowadays often sanctions such deviance by writing a generous number of allowable sick days into labour contracts.

The relationship between physicians and their patients, based as it is upon the authority of the former over the latter, is thus more than just a fortuitous consequence of doctors' professional status. It is the means to satisfaction of a need felt by many physicians to dominate others, of the need of some patients to submit before authority and of many others to acquiesce in the comfort of the structured social relations of medical care. Such habits, once acquired, are not likely to be easily abandoned so long as they fulfil a social need — notwithstanding the suggestions of some that patients should be making therapeutic decisions in particular circumstances and occasional efforts to give them an opportunity to do so.[12] In medicine as elsewhere, the tendency of many people to strive for relationships based upon authority will persevere until such time as the larger social basis for these relationships ceases to exist.

Notes

page 116: The task of drawing blood specimens is now frequently assigned to a technician specializing in that role.

page 117: Though care may suffer: patients who do not know their physicians well (and do not trust them implicitly) are less likely to comply with the necessary therapy once they have left the hospital.

page 119: Thus do we have the horrid spectacle of women who seek sterilization being talked into having unnecessary hysterectomies by residents who want the practice of removing a womb. (See J. Kozol, "A matter of life and death; the scandalous conditions at Boston City Hospital", *Ramparts*, April 1973, p48.)

page 120: Some of the more articulate patients, often thought of as troublemakers, will interrupt this elegant processional to ask questions of the physicians. These patients probably do get better care as a result, particularly on a busy ward, because they oblige the house officer to at least keep up with what is happening to them.

page 124: Even these rare exposures to the outside world are not greeted enthusiastically by academic physicians, who vote their disapproval with their feet by staying away in hordes. While Medical Mystery Tours play to packed houses every time, conferences at the Royal Victoria Hospital on such subjects as the quality of medical care are invariably poorly attended.

page 126: The cases I present in this section will be seen to be less extreme or shocking than some that have been publicized of late in the news media. I do not present extreme cases here because I think it possible, and more useful, to base an analysis on these fairly commonplace and representative examples of physician-patient interaction.

page 127: This is quite a common story. Less than a quarter of all persons with hypertension in North America are receiving adequate treatment for it, according to most surveys, in spite of the fact that many of these patients are aware that they have elevated blood pressures. A variety of "clinical judgements" and decisions are responsible for this state of affairs. (See J.A. Wilber, J.G. Barrow, "Hypertension — a community problem", *American Journal of Medicine* 52 [1972]: 652-663; E.D. Frohlich et al., "Evaluation of the initial care of hypertensive patients", *Journal of American Medical Association* 218 [1971]: 1036-1038; and S.B. Langfield, "Hypertension, deficient care of the medically served", *Annals of Internal Medicine* 78 [1973]: 19-23.)

page 128: Should such major decisions about therapy be left to the patient? Many physicians argue that confronting the patient with such data merely increases anxiety unnecessarily. As one colleague of mine put it: "How can you ask someone whether they would prefer this or that operation or this or that risk of dying? People can't make those sorts of decisions for themselves." It is certainly true that most people are not *accustomed* to making such decisions. The American sociologist Talcott Parsons agrees. He says that the tremendous gap in knowledge between the physician and the patient necessitates that the latter must trust the judgement of the former, who thus must assume the dominant position in the relationship. (See T. Parsons, *The Social System* [New York: The Free Press, 1951], pp428-479.)

That, of course, is what usually happens. It is not the only way in which physicians and patients could interact. If physicians were regarded as purveyors of information (and providers of a service), they could place a series of options regarding therapy before the patients, allowing them to make a more or less informed decision of their own. A. Cartwright, J. Lella and others have shown in an unpublished study that hospitalized patients regularly and consistently complain about lack of information from physicians. They *want* to know.

page 131: It has been shown that patients who are informed, before the operation, of the pain and discomfort they will experience afterwards, are generally able to manage their pain without analgesia (pain killers) much sooner after the operation than are patients who are not so informed. (M.S. Davis, "Variance in patients' compliance with doctors' orders: analysis of congruence between survey responses and results of empirical investigations", *Journal of Medical Education* 41 [1966]: 1037-1048).

page 132a: The demonstration of decisiveness (and this means making decisions independently of other physicians as well as of patients) is looked upon favourably as an index of the growing competence of the physician-in-training. Conversely, it is often assumed by medical school teachers that the physicians or medical students who are not very assertive are less sure of themselves. Many patients tend to judge their physicians similarly. Not all physicians systematically expropriate the patient's right to participate in decisions concerning care, of course. A small number actually do allow patients to make considered, informed and independent judgements about therapy. Others actively avoid making decisions themselves, but rather than deferring to the authority of the patient, they let another physician decide.

132b: The extent to which patients are routinely excluded from discussions about diagnosis and therapy was underlined by the recent introduction of the problem-oriented medical record-keeping system, which has become all the rage in academic hospitals. Among other things, this involves keeping track of how much patients have been told about their condition, under the heading 'patient information'. Significantly, this is included in a patient's chart *after* the articulation of diagnosis and therapy. Of course, the fact that one is keeping track of what patients know presumes that they are not to be told everything.

page 133: Thomas Szasz and Mark Hollander have delineated three patterns of physician-patient interaction. (See T.S. Szasz, M.H. Hollander, "A contribution to the philosophy of medicine", *AMA Archives of Internal Medicine* 47 [1956]: 585-592.) Eliot Friedson has suggested how these patterns are correlated with class:

[T]*he* **activity-passivity** *pattern of interaction in treatment is most likely to be found where lay culture diverges greatly from professional culture and where the status of the layman is very low compared to the professional; where the divergences are lesser, the* **guidance-co-operation** *pattern is likely to be found, whereas where both the lay culture and the status of the patient are very much like that of the profession, the* **mutual participation** *pattern is likely to be used often.* (Emphasis added.) (See E. Friedson, *Profession of Medicine, A Study of the Sociology of Applied Knowledge* [New York: Dodd Mead and Company, 1973], p321.

While these categories are rather arbitrary, they do help underline the downgrading by physicians of participation in therapy by people from lower socio-economic groups. (One physician friend of mine left his middle class environs to take over temporarily a medical practice in a working class district of Montreal. He commented that patients in this district were much more "co-operative" in accepting his diagnoses and recommendations than were his usual patients.)

page 134: Yet possibly even more important than the many pressures urging students into dominance roles is the raw material on which those pressures act — the students themselves. The special authority of physicians is so widely accepted in North American society that one can easily imagine the attractions of a medical career being particularly strong for those with a a desire to wield authority. Certainly, all medical school applicants are well aware of the phsyician's usual status in relation to patients. For most, the desire to achieve this status will have been an important criterion in their decision to seek admission.

6

Medicine on the Assembly-line

Sub-subspecialization and Technology

A friend of mine once proudly announced that he had been accepted into a very prestigious postgraduate training program in the United States, where he would be doing residencies in both cardiology and pathology.

"Why the hell would anyone want to do both?" I asked him.

"Well, I'll be able to do endomyocardial biopsies."*

"But why the pathology?"

"I'll be able to look at my own specimens under the electron microscope."

"Just for that, you'll go through a pathology residency? Isn't that a waste of manpower?"

When I pressed him a little further, he admitted that his sub-subspecialty was more a gimmick to help him get into the training program than something he really wanted to do. I later came to realize that his gravitation towards a yet unborn sub-subspecialty in which he will be the master of a little bit of technology is not an isolated phenomenon. And that he felt obliged to submit to the imperatives of technological medicine places him in much the same relationship to it as are most patients.

The parallel rise of superspecialization and supertechnology is a striking element in recent medical history and a focal point for many of the sometimes bizarre contradictions besetting the institution of medicine today. It is a development based on the largely unchallenged assumption that an increase in the sophistication of medical technology, and in the degree of specialization within the medical profession, represents an increase in the quality of health care. I hope to show in this chapter not only that our faith in this assumption is largely unfounded, but also that the assumption itself is an expression of primary forces in society.

Specialization in medicine

The notion that competent medical care can only be meted out by a specialist has become widely accepted by many North Americans.* The pressure on the medical student to become a specialist is enormous. Marcus Welby notwithstanding, specialization is the overwhelming ideology of medicine today, so much so that it can easily be forgotten that, until recently, this was not the case.

It was only with the development of antisepsis and anaesthesia late in the last century that most surgical procedures became practicable, allowing some physicians to devote their practices entirely to surgery. Not long afterwards, the "specialists" — those who claimed the most knowledge, experience and training — in nonsurgical adult medicine, the internists, declared themselves a thing apart. Even then, the bulk of medical practice remained in the hands of generalists. The American Medical Association was long an opponent of specialization; in the 1860s, it waged a bitter battle against some physicians who were interested in eye diseases and wanted to advertise as "oculists". [1]

It wasn't until the 1930s that specialization became very popular. At that time, boards were established by specialty groups in the United States to limit, through certification examination, the number of physicians entering their respective specialties.* But in spite of the establishment of these boards, specialization has been rapidly on the increase since that time, with the number of specialists increasing *eight-fold* between 1931 and 1969 while the number of general practitioners fell by more than half.*

The trend has been similar in Canada. In recent times very few medical school graduates have been entering non-specialty practice and specialists have become generally accepted as the wave of the future. The general practitioner is seen by many as a vestige of the past. Representative of this trend was the attitude of the Physician-in-Chief at one hospital I worked in. He suggested that the so-called general internists (those specialists in internal medicine who lack a *sub*specialty) should become the *primary* care practitioners of the future!

Why was there so dramatic a transition to specialty practice in the 1930s and 1940s? While the explosion of scientific knowledge in medicine was undoubtedly a necessary precondition, Rosemary Stevens, in *American Medicine and the Public Interest*, suggests that the Great Depression was a precipitating factor:

Depression conditions undoubtedly accelerated the trend. There were potential financial as well as professional advantages to the well-trained specialist to be able to hold himself out as such, whether through a special diploma, a licence, or a degree.[2]

Intense competition for patients who could pay their bills at that time combined with the availability of plentiful funding for research in medical centres[3] to make it financially worthwhile for physicians to enter specialties. Of course, all this occurred against a backdrop of continuing urbanization and the growth throughout society of increasingly large, differentiated and impersonal institutions.

The shortage of primary care practitioners is now well known. Flexner's concern that small towns were being inundated with physicians has given way to an awareness that many small towns are unable to attract any at all. By effecting the limitation of enrolment in medical schools, and by centring medical training in the university hospital, the Flexner report contributed to difficulties in obtaining the services of a general practitioner. The shortage is now almost as acute in large cities as in rural areas, compelling many people to resort to emergency rooms and to the impersonal outpatient departments of large hospitals. So great is the demand that when I finished interning, I was told that if I opened .a general practice in Montreal, it would be filled to capacity within three months.

The specialists make little effort to regulate their own numbers. Even when they appeared to be running out of patients to operate on, cardiac surgery residency programs continued to churn out new practitioners of the art.* One reason for this is that the work of specialists in hospitals is made much easier by the presence of residents and clinical fellows. To a considerable extent, the flow of physicians into specialty practice is regulated neither by the need of the community for specialists, nor by the demand upon their services, but by the never-ending need of the hospitals for residents. Hospitals need there residents, each trained in a speciality, to care for the patients of those physicians already certified as specialists.

At the same time, there has been a corresponding increase in the proportion of students who decide, at some point in their careers, to opt for a specialty, even though most are aware of the need for more general practitioners, and despite the fact that few had even begun to make up their minds on the matter at the time they began their training. My own feeling was that although I might well end up in a specialty, I certainly wasn't going to commit myself to any until I had at least sampled them all. Most of my classmates felt that way too, although there was the odd one who had "always wanted" to be a surgeon or a psychiatrist.

In spite of this, the assumption by other people that not only would we one day specialize, but that very early in medical school we should already have chosen a specialty was widespread, and demonstrates how thoroughly the idea of specialization as the *sine qua non* of good medical care has infiltrated the public mind. Of course, the expectation of outsiders that medical students will specialize is not unfounded — most do — but it is not until processing by medical schools of student raw material is well under way that the students' commitment to specialize begins to emerge. This has been convincingly documented in a study on medical specialization done by Patricia Kendall and Hanan Selvin.[4]

When they asked medical students at Cornell whether they intended to devote more of their time to specialization or to general practice, they received very different answers from the students in the early years (only one-third planned to specialize in first year) than in the later years (three-quarters of the fourth year students were heading for a specialty).*

Another study of students at the University of North Carolina showed a relatively stable minority favouring general practice, but there was a dramatic shift of those who were initially undecided into the ranks of the specialists as they progressed through medical school.[5]

Indoctrination towards specialization begins very early in medical training. As far as I can recall, I did not come into contact with a single general practitioner in a clinical setting during my entire five years of medical school and internship, and that was not because I ran away from them. I could have taken an *elective* in general practice, but like the overwhelming majority of my classmates, I did not. As astonishing as it may seem, there was no compulsory exposure in our curriculum to medical practice in a community setting.

Or hardly any. There was one exception to the medical school's general rule of placing us in the protective custody of the specialists. During the pediatrics rotation in fourth year, each student was assigned one day to visit, with a few others, a family practice in Cowansville, Quebec, about eighty miles from Montreal. None of the students who were to go on my appointed day had a car to get us there, however, so we passed it up. For many of those who did go, that half day of general practice was about all they would ever experience.*

All of our remaining clinical instruction, and much of that in the basic sciences, was given by specialists or, more precisely, by *subspecialists*. For example, we were first taught about arthritis in the context of the bizarre, fascinating immunological disorders of which arthritis can be a part, but which are only occasionally seen outside of hospital conferences and medical school classrooms. Nor was arthritis presented to us in anything like the way a practitioner would usually confront it — as a relatively common (which is to say 'uninteresting') problem whose diagnosis and treatment are reasonably straightforward.

The rare instances in which the work of general practitioners was referred to in the classroom were occasions for deriding their errors in diagnosis and therapy. Family practitioners were made out to be bumbling incompetents or, at the best of times, mere supporting actors in the high drama of the specialist's work. These prejudices were reinforced during our in-hospital training, when at least some of the patients who reached us from general practitioners (of whom there were none on staff) were the ones they had been unable to handle or had managed incorrectly.

A major complaint in almost all university hospitals I have worked in or visited is the pressure on house officers to obtain subspecialty consultations at the earliest opportunity. Many trainees express frustration at this, because they never have an opportunity to work things out for themselves. Particularly 'interesting' patients, with diseases involving several organs, are doomed to be confronted by a continuous parade of subspecialty teams (not to mention all the medical students who came sauntering by "to listen to the interesting heart in bed six").

A senior resident I worked with once remarked: "You're going to receive hundreds of consultations while you work in this hospital. I doubt if more than a handful will provide you with any useful information you didn't already have."

He was right. The subspecialists rarely told us anything we hadn't derived from a textbook or a recent article. But reluctant and sceptical as we were (at least some of the time), we usually ended up calling the consultant anyway, just to make sure we were doing things right. It is easy to understand how specialists in practice, so conditioned by their training, and without even any other house officers around to discuss a case with, lose confidence in their ability to handle problems outside their domain and refer them to other physicians.

When a cardiologist and a gastroenterologist refer patients back and forth it is reprehensible, because they should each be able to handle at least some of the problems relating to "the other's" organs. When a gynecologist and internist refer to one another, it is most fortunate: so far have they removed themselves from each other's subject-area that they probably could not approach the problems competently even if they dared try.

The prevailing ideology is that only the cardiologist *really* knows how to take care of a person with heart trouble. Others may get away with doing so, but for them it is like spitting in the dark. Likewise does the nephrologist have a monopoly on kidneys and the gastroenterologist on livers and guts. So eruditely can they articulate the differential diagnosis in even the most clear-cut case that house officers who do not call upon the appropriate consultant are bound to feel guilty.

The ethic foisted on students in the classroom, that the adequate mastery of a subject means learning everything there is to learn about it, is also gospel on the specialty wards. This is particularly true of those university hospitals (of the type in which I received most of my training) in which the specialists encountered by medical students or interns may be among the most knowledgeable in their fields. It is rarely possible to measure up to such people and trainees have no choice but to remain very humble and to get by as best they can at their relatively low level of competence until they, too, are specialists.*

In addition, the prevailing incompetence of subspecialists outside their own narrow fields encourages physicians-in-training to accept this state of affairs as the norm. When I was interning, I spent two months on a neurology ward. The two residents I worked with (one had done a year as a resident in internal medicine before entering neurology) treated me as some sort of consultant in internal medicine, because it was the area in which I was concentrating my internship. This was only three months after I had graduated from medical school!

Surgeons are particularly notorious for losing the ability to think critically about anything but surgical problems. I recall one woman who was admitted for a breast biopsy and was found to have anaemia. The surgeons decided that there were only two courses of action open to them: either to treat the patient with iron pills without trying to determine the cause of the anaemia, or to ask a haematologist to see her. They did not consider the possibility of trying to work out the cause of the anaemia for themselves by doing a few basic tests before seeking outside help.

Gynecologists are no less guilty of a one organ-system mentality. Like their surgical brethren, they become accustomed to dealing with nothing but their immediate interest. It is hardly surprising that even those who have been well trained in general medicine lose confidence in their ability to apply knowledge and skills with which they have been so long out of touch. In my experience, specialists in internal medicine are less likely to become estranged from problems and diseases that belong to other specialties, but the subspecialists among them still tend to defer to other subspecialists when another organ system is in question.

One nearly universal tendency among internists is to steer clear of the gynecologist's territory when doing an otherwise general examination. When I was a fourth-year student, my resident and I decided to do a pelvic examination on a patient who was rather ill with an infection from an unknown source, and whose condition precluded our waiting for a consultant. There were no facilities for doing a pelvic on the ward where we were working, so we took the patient to another ward. We found an examining table there, but no equipment to use for the examination. After running about the hospital for half the evening, we were finally able to examine her; clearly, pelvics were not encouraged!

That physicians can only feel comfortable within the confines of a specialty is largely a function of attitudes they acquired relatively early in their training. Medical schools would have their students believe that the way to approach diagnosis and treatment is the way articulated weekly in the *New England Journal of Medicine*. Its regularly-featured 'clinical-pathological conference', mentioned earlier, usually concerns a patient with a bizarre disease and is always discussed by someone who is expert (to the point of renown) in the relevant field. This expert is supposed to know all there is to know and then some about the differential diagnosis of the case presented, including all the latest studies and speculations, right down to the most improbable syndromes.

The strong implication for student physicians is that doctors can only deal with a problem effectively when they can talk about it exhaustively and eruditely. We learned to see disease through the eyes of a series of specialists. That which interested our teachers came to be challenging and interesting for us. That which bored them (many of the mundane problems which make up the bulk of medical practice) was not likely to stimulate the class. The style of medical practice to which we were exposed was the one which prevailed in the teaching hospital: physicians performing life-saving interventions in medical emergencies; investigators solving complicated diagnostic problems, practitioners ordering countless tests in the hope of uncovering the unexpected (but always hoped-for) Big Diagnosis; and specialists performing recitals of every aspect of a disease and of every contingency that might arise, hardly ever referring to a book. We learned to be turned on to the exotic disease rather than to the average patient: in short, we were encouraged to become everything that the general practitioner was not.

According to Kendall and Selvin:

[A]s these students learn more in medical school, they come to recognize both the vast complexities of modern medicine and their own limitations in being able to cope with all these complexities effectively. As a result of this new-found awareness, they feel compelled to select a particular field in which to develop their competence. [6]

Many students do develop such a perspective, but it is difficult to justify. It was the Flexner Report that welded the education of the medical student to the university teaching hospital. Few would suggest that what students are exposed to in this setting is very representative of medical practice, and some are coming to believe that it is not even a very good place to obtain a medical education. [7]

Working on the wards of the hospital (they are *specialty* wards, of course) is not an experience that can be taken lightly. When students complete a rotation on a ward, they often leave with a feeling of inadequacy in the face of the tremendous knowledge that the subspecialists possess — in their subspecialty. [8]

One consequence of the degree of differentiation of specialists is that they can often be heard to talk contemptuously of one another's specialties. The internist derides the clinical knowledge and judgement of the surgeon; the latter is disdainful in return. (One popular expression of their mutual antagonism is "the internist knows everything and does nothing, while the surgeon knows nothing and does everything.") The general practitioner is even more the butt of irreverent jokes from the specialists, a fact pointedly obvious to house officers and medical students. (The classic formulation here is "the specialist knows more and more about less and less, while the general practitioner knows less and less about more and more".)

It is undeniably true that many general practitioners do not practise well, but that is not to say they are incapable of doing so. Many are unable to spend enough time with their patients, either because of the great demand on their services or because they want to process as many people as possible in order to maximize their incomes. Nor, in a fee-for-service arrangement, is there any incentive for them to 'keep up' by taking the time to read medical journals.

In Britain, where the evolution of the medical profession has been very different, the general practitioner has an important place in the care of all citizens. Long before specialization became the dominant trend in North American medicine, the British had seen a division of practitioners into surgeons (originally barbers), physicians, and apothecaries (dispensers of medicaments). Their present health care system perpetuates a tripartite profession of general practitioners (who deliver primary care), surgeons and physicians (the latter two groups being exclusively consultants). No one except the wealthy (who can afford to see practitioners working outside the National Health Service) can go to a specialist without the advice of a general practitioner, and no one has to go to a hospital clinic to receive their primary care.[9]

The flow of British medical school graduates into specialty practice is carefully regulated by the National Health Service, and the great majority of physicians in Britain are not specialists. If graduates wish, they may receive *some* specialized postgraduate training, but the number of appointments to specialty posts in hospitals is very limited, and the acquisition of such a post is a prerequisite to specialty practice.[10]

Are the British receiving inferior care because of their relative lack of specialists? Objective data on health status on both sides of the Atlantic (like life expectancy, and maternal and infant mortality figures), indicate that their health care is as good as that in the United States and Canada.[11]

Is there anything wrong with the care delivered by specialists? Certain data published recently indicate that there is. When rates of certain surgical procedures per unit population in Canada and Great Britain are compared, it is found that operations such as cholecystectomy (removal of the gall bladder), hysterectomy (removal of the uterus), appendectomy and tonsillectomy are being performed much more frequently in Canada *where there are more surgeons.*[12] It is not possible to explain this difference on the basis of a greater prevalence in Canada of diseases in the organs involved.

Besides such disturbing indications of unnecessary interventions on the part of specialists, it is doubtful that a health care system so top-heavy with specialists will be able to deal adequately with mundane but important disorders such as hypertension. The tendency in North America in recent years has been to train technicians and nurses to handle problems that are felt to be insufficiently complex for physicians.[13]

There is one remaining aspect of the trend to specialization that should be discussed. Granted that physicians want to have specialized knowledge, why do they feel they must be *certified* as competent in their specialties by the profession? The reasons are complex. In some places, but not all, it is necessary for physicians to be certified as specialists before they can admit patients to certain hospitals and perform operations upon them there. Frequently, physicians can earn more for certain medical acts if they have specialty certification. Still, there are many situations in which physicians can practise as specialists without a certificate (surgeons and ophthalmologists working in association with community hospitals or in small towns, for example, and internists in most situations). Of course, they benefit handsomely from the status of specialty certification once it is achieved. By rising through the ranks they "earn" the right to pre-eminence in the consumer society, to a superior position not only in their encounters with patients but in all their social and economic relations.*

The game of graded promotions is at least partly responsible for the intensely-felt need to be certified. Physicians are indoctrinated to the belief that competence is proportional to rank and that certification of progress is necessary at each stage. The idea of entering practice before being pronounced fit to do so is alien to and incompatible with much that physicians have been taught.* This comes back to the problem of authority: physicians-in-training submit before the exaggerated authority of their superiors as part and parcel of their acceptance of the authority of the specialty certificate and the structured programme through which it can be obtained. This submission is also consistent with their preference for relationships with others that are likewise based on authority.

A surgical resident in Montreal committed suicide recently upon learning that he had failed his certification examination. That certification can matter so much surely suggests that the certificate means more to physicians-in-training than a little extra money. Self-esteem is on the line when residents set out in search of specialty papers. Continually confronted with evidence of their own relative incompetence, they are led to believe that only when they are certified will they have any skill worth mentioning.

Modern medical technology

There is now and probably always has been widespread enthusiasm for the evolving contribution of technology to the field of medical care. The many potential benefits of the new technological medicine have been catalogued in a book by David Rutstein.[14] He discusses machines that save and preserve lives as well as looking at the computer as a labour-saving device and aid to more efficient research. The Program on Technology and Society at Harvard University has singled out medicine as an area that exemplifies what good technology can do:

[Recent advances] have created two new opportunities: (1) they have made possible treatments and cures that were never possible before, and (2) they provide a necessary condition for the delivery of adequate medical care to the population at large as a matter of right rather than of privilege.[15]

The Big Machine arrived at the Montreal Neurological Institute while I was rotating through there during my internship. It was known as an EMI-scanner (for Electronic Musical Instruments Co., which developed the device after it stopped producing Beatles records). The machine's generic name is CT-scanner (for computed tomography). It is used for the x-ray examination of the brain and has already revolutionized neuroradiology. It allows for more specific determination of what is going on inside someone's head than does any other diagnostic procedure, save a few that are more dangerous and often painful.

The CT-scanner we received was only the third to be installed in North America, and the waiting list for the machines was said to be several years long. The story of how the Institute was able to be one of the first to get one is rather interesting. The Director of the Institute, a neurosurgeon, was in England at the time that the first rumours were leaked about the pending availability of the $350,000 toys. With some fancy footwork, he found out where and how they could be obtained and (so the story goes) he placed an order for one without even obtaining prior authorization for the expense. Presumably, he knew that this was a piece of hardware no board of directors could possibly turn down.

The arrival of the Big Machine was greeted with the sort of festivities that in another era might have accompanied the launching of an oceanliner. Not only was it thought to be a valuable addition to the diagnostic armamentarium, but it was also something no other hospital in the country had, at least for the time being, and it was bound to augment the MNI's prestige.

Only one of the neurologists seemed at all sceptical. "I want to see it in action first," he said. "No machine can do the work of a good clinician, but the way people are talking about this one, it is supposed to make the medical history and the physical examination obsolete."

I saw him again a year later. "I've beaten the machine three times already," he told me. "You can't accept these data uncritically, but many people seem prepared to do so."

At the time of writing this book, several other CT-scanners have already been installed across Canada. Although no reports have yet appeared in the medical literature indicating that CT-scanning has an effect on the outcome of medical care,[16] as of April, 1977, 567 of the machines had been installed throughout the United

States (entailing an annual technical and professional cost of more than $280 million), with another 283 on the way.[17] Many university hospitals now have two scanners, one for heads and one for bodies, and for some, even that is not enough.* There is no doubt that these machines are a valuable diagnostic tool in neurology. Unfortunately, they are now being used on many people with minor neurologic problems, people who don't need them. They have to be used in this way, however, if they are to "pay their way".

These machines were not introduced against a background of unlimited funding. The same month that the CT-scanner arrived in Montreal, the resident staff of one hospital in town was told that they could not have an electrocardiograph machine on every ward "because they cost $925 each".

Of course, the technological innovations in modern medicine do not all require a capital investment of hundreds of thousands of dollars; Big Technology consists of many small items as well. A case in point is a machine that can be found in the biochemistry laboratory of almost every hospital, large or small, throughout North America. This device is the 'SMA-12' autoanalyser', and it is capable of automatically measuring the quantities of twelve chemicals in a given blood sample.

This sounds ideal for mass screening for disease, and the test is very popular with physicians. I have only worked in one hospital where it was not routine procedure to do an SMA-12 on *every* patient on admission and, frequently, several more times during hospitalization. One would hope that doing this would occasionally uncover unexpected diseases, leading to life-saving treatment. Unfortunately, it doesn't work out that way. A recent study of routine admission blood tests showed that the machines hardly ever turn up an unexpected diagnosis. If physicians ordered only those tests that seemed to be called for in a particular situation (by the history and physical findings), they might well accomplish just as much diagnostically.[18]

Some consequences of the use of the SMA-12 can be detrimental to patient care. The SMA-12, like other machines, can give inaccurate results. At the Royal Victoria Hospital, we were always running into erroneously elevated values of an enzyme called alkaline phosphatase. This enzyme is increased in the presence of certain diseases of liver and bone. Particularly when cancer spreads to bone, 'alk. phos.' goes up. I can't begin to count the number of times that I have kept patients in the hospital for needless, extended investigations in the search for cancers they did not have, just because they had reported elevations in alkaline phosphatase.

One thing we never did when chasing the cause of the high enzyme reading was consider the suggestion of the distinguished British epidemiologist Archie Cochrane: "Before ordering a test, decide what you will do if it is (a) positive, or (b) negative, and if both answers are the same don't do the test."[19] Even when the source of an elevated alkaline phosphatase is found, rarely is anything done about it in a person who is without symptoms. By the time a cancer has spread to bone, cure is not possible and relief of symptoms is the principal consideration guiding a choice of therapy.

In spite of lack of evidence of its usefulness, the SMA-12 test is firmly embedded in clinical practice, and is performed hundreds of times daily, at considerable cost, in the typical major metropolitan hospital.

All cautionary examples notwithstanding, however, the trend to technologize proceeds apace, led, one feels, by those whose critical faculties have atrophied under the spell of the shiny new machines. A particularly goggle-eyed endorsement of technological innovations in medicine appeared in an *Atlantic Monthly* article by Jerry Avorn, a graduate of Harvard Medical School.[20] Avorn outlined a scenario for a future in which the role of computers in patient care will have greatly increased. As he sees it, computers will take care of much of the patient interviews and examinations, the diagnosing of disease and the institution of treatment. The computers in turn would nominally be under the control of physicians, physicians' assistants and patients.

Avorn also foresees what I suppose will have to be designated a 'primary care computer', programmed to "express sympathy for patients suffering from particular symptoms or relief that a given organ has been producing no complaints." Furthermore, Avorn suggests that the computer could bridge that troublesome linguistic, educational and cultural barrier between physicians and so many of their patients by determining "the language and level most appropriate for the patient and then [turning] itself onto the proper program."[21]

Reductio ad absurdum, it would seem, for Avorn's brave new world, but he should perhaps be excused for thinking as he does. He admits that during his time as a student at the Massachusetts General Hospital, he got along better with the teaching machines than he did with human instructors. The prospect is nonetheless disturbing, because he is far from being alone in his view of what the future of medical care should be.[22]

The consequences of technology in medicine

The rise of the hospital as the centre of medical care has led to the concentration of capital in single, large institutions, which in turn has created the necessary base for technological medicine. Super-technology can only exist in centres where there are sufficient specialists to ensure that it will be utilized to the maximum, and hence efficiently. But just because there are enough physicians around to keep a machine busy does not mean that it will only be acquired when the priorities of the community call for it. Some technology, like that surrounding coronary care, is acquired because there has been an artificial need (independent of its true worth) generated for it in the community because its razzle-dazzle is thought to reflect the quality of care that an institution should be delivering.

Cardiac surgery equipment, as a particularly high-profile embodiment of technological medicine in our time, is another commodity that hospitals use to enhance their prestige and that becomes an end in itself, a substitute for health care. Since cardiac surgery equipment is so very expensive, it would make sense economically to limit it to a small number of centres, but few hospitals want to admit that they aren't important enough to have this machinery. That most community hospitals now have facilities for some heart surgery has led to tragic consequences, since the mortality rates for complicated procedures are generally higher in the smaller centres. Some experts have suggested that fewer patients would die if these procedures were only done in a small number of centres, since they would inevitably be under the care of more experienced surgeons.[23]

Adding to the cost of technological development is the highly specialized technical work force that comes with it. Each technological innovation adds one, two or even three new types of hospital workers. Not too many years ago, the electrocardiography technician was the only specialized worker in the cardiology department (and, lest we forget, even the electrocardiogram is a relatively recent development). When the CT-scanner came to the Montreal Neurological Institute, so did two technicians, because it could only be operated by people who had taken a special training program in England. Many hospital laboratories have machines that can be operated by only one technician, working full-time on that one machine. Such division of labour means, among other things, that when these people are not in the hospital, their equipment cannot be used.

The hospital of Florence Nightingale (and even that of Dr. Kildare), which consisted largely of physicians and nurses, no longer exists. Nurses are still the largest occupational category within a hospital, but physicians are being overtaken in numbers by the technical staff. Physicians have increasingly become specialized in their orientation, subspecialized in expertise (which is limited to one organ or organ system) and sub-subspecialized in the application of a particular bit of technology to their subspecialty. A brigade of hospital workers has become the technical support staff for any one sub-subspecialty.

These technical workers are so scattered throughout the hospital that solidarity and a sense of common purpose are often unrealizable among them. There is not necessarily even any contact among technicians working within one specialty department (as, for example, with the neurologically oriented technical staff who deal with CT-scanning, brain scanning and electroencephalography). In their isolation, they are easily exploited: hospital technicians are frequently paid much less than workers with comparable skills in private industry, and they are discouraged from striking because of the "essential services" they are providing.

Technicians rarely meet a particular patient more than once or twice, and there is scarcely an opportunity for human contact to develop. This leads to estrangement, both for the patients, who are always being processed by persons they hardly know, if at all (including many of the physicians), and for the technicians, who are too busy turning their screws on the hospital assembly line to be able to relate to the people passing through their cubicles. Some technicians never even get to see the patients who are the presumed focus of their endeavours.

People who come to the emergency room of a hospital with a diagnosed or suspected heart attack are generally admitted to the Coronary Care Unit (CCU). In consideration for the remote possibility that the patient might die on the way to the CCU, an intern or resident usually comes along on this fateful journey. When I worked in Emergency as an intern, this was one of my responsibilities. With a syringe full of lidocaine in hand (to reverse any cardiac arrest), I would roll the bed down the corridors feeling ten feet tall. There is considerable drama surrounding the care of the coronary patient, and the exciting run from the emergency room is an appropriate introduction to the high technology of the CCU.

Hospitals crawl all over one another these days in the search for more sophisticated monitoring equipment, in the reasonable belief that anything that might detect a potentially fatal arrhythmia and allow life-saving treatment is worth any price. The Royal Victoria was one of the first hospitals to establish a CCU in the 1950s but when I interned there the equipment was, by latter-day standards, hopelessly out of date. They were still using much of their original equipment; I have seen fancier machinery in a small hospital in Claxton, Georgia. The sophistication of machinery in some university hospitals is staggering: computer analyses of the heart rhythm, instant replays on demand of the electrocardiograph pattern for the previous thirty seconds, simultaneous transmission of the electrocardiograph to monitors at the patient's bedside and at the nursing station and more. All the Royal Vic had was a simple bedside monitor: if a patient disturbed the electrodes installed on his or her chest (by moving, for example), a buzzer would go off, indicating a possible cardiac arrest. A nurse would run to the patient's room and see if it was a false alarm (as it was 99 per cent of the time) or a real cardiac arrest.

As surprising as it may seem, this "obsolete" unit had very good results in terms of patient survival, and some cardiology fellows told me that it was precisely the lack of sophisticated equipment which was responsible for the unit's good track record. When hospitals use remote monitors, at a nursing station for instance, the patterns on the screen are open to a number of interpretations. But at the Royal Vic, when nurses had to run to their patients' bedsides to see what was happening, they would be able to determine more quickly whether a cardiac arrest had in fact taken place. This, of course, did not deter the Royal Vic from acquiring some of the fancier stuff. Now no physician there need feel ashamed of the quality of the equipment in the CCU.

Sophisticated equipment or otherwise, no CCU buff greeted very enthusiastically a report in the *British Medical Journal* by H.G. Mather and his colleagues, a report which has cast considerable doubt on the value of *any* coronary care unit. The authors randomly picked persons with uncomplicated myocardial infarctions (heart attacks) and either sent them home to rest in bed, or, like the usual practice, into a CCU. Notwithstanding the fact that many people considered this controlled trial unethical (it would "deny" coronary care to people who "obviously" would benefit from it), it turned out that there was a lower mortality rate in the group sent home than among those admitted to CCUs. The reason for this anomalous result is presumably that the anxiety of being in the hospital, coupled with the sometimes morbid effects of technological interventions, causes the deaths of more patients than all the devices of modern medicine can save.[24] Much to the consternation of many cardiologists who rejected this report, a second study once again failed to demonstrate an advantage for the CCU over home care in treatment of these patients.*[25]

Yet technological innovations in medicine have been, for instance, largely responsible for the growth of sub-subspecialties within the now familiar subspecialties of cardiology, nephrology, and neurology. In the ranks of cardiologists can now be found those who sub-subspecialize in echocardiography (an adaptation of radar), angiocardiography (injecting dye into the heart to examine its blood vessels) and phonocardiography (a special method of recording the sounds of heart valves).* Most physicians no longer even try to fathom all the technology to which they are daily submitting their patients; they settle, instead, for mastering a small part of it and resign themselves to being intimidated and mystified by the rest. Almost every time I attended a cardiology conference in a hospital, I was swamped with data I could barely grasp, if at all, from sophisticated machines that were fascinating to cardiologists, but not of much practical value to house officers like myself. Physicians can even be intimidated by technicians, who might take the chance to show off their highly specialized knowledge while explaining the significance of a particular patient's results.

It would be a mistake, then, to regard the development of a technological medicine as exclusively an idealistic effort on the part of some to provide better medical care to all. The phenomenon clearly results in part from the internal dynamics of the medical profession — the specialization and increasing concentration in "centres of medical excellence" — but this is only one of the forces.* Another force, as Eliot Krause has observed, lies in the corporations involved in the manufacture and marketing of the devices themselves.[25] Like other corporations, Krause points out, these are primarily interested in profits.[26] Furthermore, the medical marketplace, like that for military technology, often operates as a monopoly or a near-monopoly. Some authors describe a medical-industrial complex, which generates needs for the products of the extremely prosperous medical technology sector and which is increasingly the domain of large corporations:

[T]he aim of the health industry is not to promote the general health and well-being (that would be self-defeating), but to exploit profitable markets and to create new ones. The emphasis, then, is not on products and services which would improve basic health care for the great mass of consumers, but on what are essentially luxury items: computerized equipment for intensive cardiac care units, hyperbaric chambers, etc. Under the pressure of the industry's barrage of packaged technology, the delivery system is increasingly distorted towards high-cost, low-utilization inpatient services.[27]

The evolution of medical technology manufacturing is quite

typical of big business monopolies. Many of the larger corporations initially involved in the production of one type of medical product have been branching out in a vertical and horizontal integration of the manufacture and distribution of different kinds of medical hardware and software. They are even getting into the business of designing and building hospitals. Thus, yesterday's baby powder producer becomes today's manufacturer of medications. Thus, too, is the leading manufacturer of prescription pharmaceuticals in the United States a conglomerate called American Home Products.[28]

Like their counterparts in other sectors of the economy, medically-oriented corporations seek to create a need for their products, be they medications or sophisticated machines,[29] and they peddle their wares even when they know them to be dangerous.* Corporations in the medical sector of the economy are unusual in only one respect: they do much better than other industries, realizing an annual rate of profit of twenty per cent of investment. This handsome return comes from the consuming public, both directly (in the sale of prescription drugs) and indirectly (in the form of machinery that continues to escalate health care costs).[30]

A third force that has done much to promote technological growth comes from the communities where hospitals are located, and where the availability of high-powered technology often seems to be a major concern. Once, while leafing through a world almanac at a newstand, I turned to the entry on my home town of Winnipeg. In the half-dozen lines allotted, the item made a point of describing Winnipeg as a major medical centre, where important medical research was being done in the area of immunology. This had a certain irony for me, because I had worked during one of my medical school elective periods for the Manitoba government on the preparation of a working paper on health care priorities. According to that document, the concentration of health care expenditures in hospital facilities in the metropolis was one of the major problems of the system, resulting in rapid escalation in the cost of medical care and in inequitable distribution of resources among the population.[31]

The paper proposed that this problem could be alleviated by decentralizing care, establishing a network of community clinics and allowing for the rational and integrated distribution of the machines of the new technology throughout the province. Needless to say, this did not go over too well with the university physicians, who were not pleased at the prospect of having the number of hospital beds reduced. 'Private enterprisers' and their media allies condemned the proposed innovations as well, considering them to be inconsistent with "freedom of choice" in the selection of medical care services. Much of the public, so indoctrinated in the ideology of the modern technological medicine, also stood opposed.

Expensive technological medicine need not interfere with good medical care. However, some serious students of medical technology have raised the question of whether or not the miracle machines have *any value at all:*

Most of the electronic devices and computerized systems that have been tried are sophisticated, unreliable, hard to use, and extremely expensive. There is little reason to believe, considering all their side effects, that they save the physician much time and effort. [32]

In spite of such analyses, and the admonitions of the renowned British epidemiologist, Dr. A.L. Cochrane, and others, [33] it seems improbable that there will be a diminution in the role of technology in North American medicine, so much is it a part of our conception of what health care is supposed to be. [34] But the rise of technology and the concomitant specialization of the work force are not peculiar to medicine; both phenomena are prevalent throughout society.

Lewis Mumford, a prolific commentator on the problems raised by technology, suggests that society has now become what he terms a "megamachine". He argues that technology is responsible for many social ills, including turning people into "things". He assumes that the negative effects of technology operate independently of the society in which it is used, that there can be no society in which these effects will not be present. [35]

Karl Marx, on the other hand, who perceived better than most in his time the role technology was beginning to play, argues that it is only in the specific situation of a capitalist social and economic world order, in which the means of production are not in the control of the workers, that technology will be put to inhumane uses:

[With the system of private property] every man speculates on creating a new need in another in order to force him into a new sacrifice, to place him in a new dependence and to entice him into a new kind of pleasure and thereby into economic ruin. [36]

Marx also talks about the role of technology in compounding alienation:

[T]he production of too many useful things produces too large a useless population . . . The machine accommodates itself to the weaknesses of the human being in order to make the weak human being into a machine . . . The increase in the quantity of objects is accompanied by an extension of the realm of alien powers to which man is subjected, and every new product represents a new possibility of mutual swindling and mutual plundering. Man becomes ever poorer as man . . . [37]

Research scientists are acting in accordance with alienated needs when they wield equipment which, more than anything else, permits them to play in the big leagues of academia.[38] Physicians who subscribe to the idea that machines can do a better job of relating to patients, or who prescribe psychotropic drugs, such as tranquilizers, to save themselves the trouble of working through a problem with a patient, are expressing an alienated relationship to other people. Similarly, the business executives who provide the technology, by speculating on how they can create new needs in others and place them in new dependencies, are also expressing an alienated need: to extract a profit from their interaction with others. All of these phenomena are typical of our society, but it is nevertheless possible to envision a society where these alienated needs and relations would not exist and where the uses to which all technology is put would be neither inhumane nor wasteful.

Marx gives a clue to the answer when he says, "In practice I can only relate myself in a human way to a thing when the thing is related in a human way to man."[39] Humanization of technology is conceivable in a situation in which one's relation to the environment is no longer alienated.* This, of course, is only possible given the transcendance of all alienated social relations, which in turn means a larger transformation of the social and economic order.

In the meantime, the consumer benefits only occasionally from the overbearing presence of technological medicine. While it would be quite inappropriate to detechnologize medicine,* we must recognize that the most consistent effect of medical technology at present is to make both patients and health workers more passive in the delivery of medical care.

The situation is unhealthy, but this pattern of development will not be arrested merely by legislating an end to the proliferation of sub-subspecialties or by limiting the expenditures on technological medicine, or even by eliminating the profit motive from the process of production. Some societies have attempted to implement such changes from above but have been less than wholly successful in stemming the strong tendency of physicians to specialize and to work in centres that possess Big Technology.[40] The primacy of technology, in medicine as elsewhere, is a predictable function of alienated relations in modern society. Only when the transformation of the social and economic order enables a transcendance of this alienation can we expect trends in technological medicine and in medical specialization to assume human proportions and to conform to real human needs. Then it will happen not by fiat, but as a matter of course.

Notes

page 139: An endomyocardial biopsy is a procedure in which a biopsy specimen is taken through a catheter inserted into the heart.

page 140a: Nor are other nations or ideologies immune from such beliefs. No less a person than V.I. Lenin, who claimed to be an advocate of social change, wrote the following to a friend upon learning that the friend was receiving medical care from a fellow Bolshevik:

God save you from doctor-comrades in general, and doctor-Bolsheviks in particular! But really, in 99 cases out of 100, doctor-comrades are asses . . . I assure you that except in trivial cases, one should be treated only by men of first-class reputation. (V.I. Lenin, "Letter to Gorky, Nov. 1913"; quoted in B. Wolfe, *Three Who Made a Revolution,* [New York: Dial Press, 1964] p613.)

140b: Once the trend was established in 1930 with an American Board of Obstetrics, everyone else followed suit: dermatology (1932), pediatrics (1933), radiology, psychiatry and neurology, orthopedic surgery, colon and rectal surgery (1934), urology (1935), pathology, internal medicine (1936), anaesthesiology, plastic surgery, surgery (1937), neurosurgery (1940). (See "Health Manpower Source Book", Section 14: Medical Specialists, table 6, in *Journal of American Medical Association* 114 [1940]: 1663; quoted in R. Stevens, *American Medicine and the Public Interest* [New Haven: Yale University Press, 1971], p542.)

140c: Here are the figures:

	1931	1940	1949	1960	1963	1969
Full-time specialists	24,826	36,880	62,688	114,578	145,983	193,628
Part-time specialists and general practitioners	120,399	120,090	110,441	85,278	77,229	57,522

(From R. Stevens, *op.cit.,* p181.)

page 141: The procedure that has become the bread and butter of cardiac surgeons, the coronary artery bypass graft, has been under attack of late, because it has not been demonstrated to prolong life — one of the main reasons for performing it — except in a readily-defined minority of the patients. The principal, well-controlled study that demonstrated this (M.L. Murphy, H.N. Hultgren, K. Detre et al., "Treatment of Chronic Stable Angina. A preliminary report of survival data of the randomized Veterans Administration Cooperative Study", *New England Journal of Medicine* 297 (1977): 621-627) has been condemned by almost all the surgeons who have commented on it publicly or in print, while many nonsurgeons have praised it. One prominent cardiologist has expressed concern that the demand which this operation has created for additional trained heart surgeons and other personnel may resist all efforts to cut it down to size as the indications for the procedure become clearly defined and limited: "This rapidly growing enterprise is developing a momentum and a constituency of its own, and as time passes, it will be progressively more difficult and costly to curtail it materially, if the results of carefully designed studies of its efficacy prove this step to be necessary." (See E. Brunwald, "Coronary artery surgery at the crossroads", *New England Journal of Medicine* 297 [1977]: 661-663.)

page 142a: The breakdown was as follows:

	1st year students	2nd year students	3rd year students	4th year students
General practice	60%	56%	39%	16%
Specialty practice	35%	41%	56%	74%
Other	10%	5%	3%	5%

(research and teaching)

(P.L. Kendall, H.C. Selvin, "Tendencies toward specialization in medical training", in R.K. Merton, G.C. Reader and P.L. Kendall [eds].* *The Student Physician* [Cambridge, Mass.: Harvard University Press, 1957] pp153-176.)

142b: This situation was not unique to McGill. Kendall (cited above) has discussed the tendency of many medical centres to keep education of students a preserve of the specialists.

page 144: Predictably, the proportion of students who end up in specialties is highest in these "high-powered" medical centres where the role models of the superspecialists are overwhelming. (See C.N. Theodore, G.E. Sutter, J.N. Haug, *Medical School Alumni, 1967* [Chicago: American Medical Association, 1968], Table 4, pp222-312.)

page 148a: This is ironic, considering how recent a development in North American medicine the specialty boards are. In fact, there are still many specialists around who, having entered into practice before the boards existed, never had to take a certification examination.

148b: Physicians are perhaps wise to play along in the game of graded promotions. If they did not they would be hard pressed to justify a system of medical care delivery that denies access to the tools to practise medicine, however straightforward the problem to be solved, to all but the select few who call themselves physicians.

page 150: The rapid proliferation of these enormously expensive machines in the last four years has caused some alarm amongst health planners who fear that the cost of health care will skyrocket while a few reap enormous profits. (See S.H. Shapiro, S.M. Wyman, "CAT Fever", *New England Journal of Medicine* 294 [1976]: 954-956.)

page 154: Technology can even have adverse effects upon research endeavours. The respiratory diseases division at the Royal Vic is renowned for its work. It was quite a surprise for me to learn from a resident working there that much of their equipment was inferior to that of some other centres. Commented the resident: "The reason why they've produced so much good research is just because they don't have the fancy equipment. They have to be innovative and figure things out for themselves."

page 155a: Other sub-subspecialties of cardiology include adult congenital heart disease, cardiac electrophysiology, exercise testing, coronary care and electrocardiography. Medical students have long been obliged to face the inevitable cocktail patter: "Yes, but what are you going to *do?*" In other words, in what are you going to specialize? Alas, this is no longer enough. Sub-subspecialization is now sufficiently the rule that even the fellow in cardiology is often confronted with the same question.

155b: Proximity to one of these "centres of medical excellence" does not guarantee good medical care; the central Montreal community is full of hospitals, including a number of university hospitals, but the citizens who live there do not often get to reap the fruits of this harvest. In the words of Krause:

[M]*edical technology is not sold in a vacuum; it is bought. Perhaps those most interested in technological advances are the research physicians in university teaching hospitals. Both scientific curiosity and the desire for rapid career advancement through "frontier research" dictate their position on the apportionment of the hospital budget: support the research group and the hospital will become famous as an advanced medical centre . . . "Advanced technology" in medicine has prestige value and news or public relations value. Research physicians, for genuinely altruistic reasons, for scientific reasons, and for self-oriented reasons — and usually for a combination of all three — form a strong pro-technology interest group in most hospitals, especially in major medical centres.* (E. Krause, "Health and the politics of technology", *Inquiry* 8, no.3 [1971]: 54.)

page 156: Parke, Davis and Company did this with the antibiotic chloramphenicol. (See S. Sesser, "Peddling dangerous drugs abroad — special dispensation", *New Republic,* March 16, 1971, pp16-17.)

page 158a: It is important to note that Marx only described a new product as a *possibility* for deceit and robbery. That possibility is realized in capitalist society, in which people (alienated in relations to their labour, to the product of their labour and to others around them) attempt to exploit others to fulfil the needs they experience within that society. Thus is Marx's analysis quite different from that of Mumford, who would lay the blame on technology itself.

Some authors have interpreted Marx's writings as suggesting that productive technology is responsible for all other developments in society. This "technological determinism" does not withstand critical scrutiny, as Bertell Ollman points out:

It does not require a profound knowledge of history to see that technological development is variably a function of the level of science, the laws of a country, the politics of a regime, consumer demand, and much else. Thus, technology is obviously dependent in numerous important ways on the character and changes occurring in those areas of life which it is supposed to determine [according to the theory of the technological determinists].

Ollman suggests that the mode of production (productive technology) be placed in an appropriate perspective in the context of people's alienated social relations:

[I]*nstead of seeking a strict causal tie between the mode of production and other institutions and practices of society which precludes complex social interaction, we must begin by accepting the existence of this interaction and then seek out the ways in which Marx believes that the effects proceeding from the mode of production and other economic factors (narrowly understood) are more important.* (B. Ollman, *Alienation: Marx's Conception of Man in Capitalist Society*, [Cambridge University Press, 1971], pp 7-8 and 26.)

The proposals some people have made for uses of computers in medicine are expressions of humanity's condition in the society in which we live:

The possibility that we can build robots who are like men belongs, if anywhere, to the future. But the present already shows us men who act like robots. When the majority of men are like robots, then indeed there will be no problem in building robots who are like men. The idea of a manlike computer is a good example of the alternative between the human and inhuman uses of the machine. The computer can serve the enhancement of life in many respects. But the idea that it replaces man and life is the manifestation of the pathology of today. (E. Fromm, *The Revolution of Hope: Towards a Humanized Technology* [New York, Harper and Row, 1968], p46.)

158b: Where would we be without penicillin and antihypertensive medications, for example?

7

Doctor Talk

The Jargon of Medicine

Like most other institutions in society, medicine has its share of holy places. The operating room, the kitchen in the house staff residence and certain tables in the hospital cafeteria immediately spring to mind: these are places where only the duly initiated, qualified, and certified feel comfortable, where the outsider feels lost.

The medical library is another such spot. In the library, although entrance is not barred to all non-physicians, it is in fact only the physicians and their proteges who can, by making some sense of the literature, really penetrate the intrigue, and the hidden meanings, of the place. For me, going to the library as a medical student was a new and particularly exhilarating experience: the thrill, for instance, of being able to thumb through a medical journal, feeling that simply being able to do that was part of my vocation and a measure of my maturity. In a way the feeling was comparable to the male pubescent experience of devouring pornographic magazines on the newsstands of drug stores. Both experiences provide the thrill that comes from unlocking a treasure trove previously forbidden, whose significance you do not even yet fully appreciate.

The problems of delving into the medical literature are a basic difficulty in grasping the meaning of much of the vocabulary used and the resultant inability to understand the issues being discussed. Needless to say, knowing medical jargon, which is technical and highly specific to the field, is a prerequisite to any comprehension of what is written in the journals or textbooks.

Technical jargon

Before physicians can begin to use the technical lexicon of medicine, they must, of course, learn it. During an early meeting of my medical class in first year, we were promised a five thousand word increase in our vocabularies within the year. Learning those words turned out to be a tedious process and unhappily, many of them were of little use later on in our studies and in medical practice. As we went along we discovered that learning names for parts of the body and details of bodily processes does not contribute much to the comprehension of medical literature, which deals principally with diseases and their treatments. On the final day of first-year examinations, our brains were cluttered with names and formulae that, as more than one student remarked, we would never again know quite so well.

Second year brought us to a new level of understanding. Our biology of disease course introduced the language of pathology and microbiology, building blocks of the medical literature we so wanted to be able to read. Some members of the class began subscribing to the *New England Journal of Medicine* at that time. Some remarked that they were beginning to "feel like doctors" now that they could at last begin to comprehend the literature.

Our grasp of the jargon was not yet complete, however; in second year we still had to learn the vocabularies of clinical medicine and then pharmacology, which is taught a little later in the course at McGill than elsewhere. I did not subscribe to the *NEJM* that year, but I did peruse it in the library occasionally. Even then, I found much of the terminology obscure. I was not able to feel at ease with it, as it turned out, until I had completed the pharmacology course in third year.

By the time we emerged from the classroom and "hit the wards" in third and fourth years, we were well-endowed with medical terminology, if somewhat uncomfortable about using it. In those last two years of medical school, no journal was too tough a nut to crack (conversations with physicians were something else), and the medical library was like a home away from home.

Attaining proficiency in complex, technical vocabulary goes back again to Abraham Flexner's "scientific basis of medical practice". Of course, medicine has become much more complex in the years since the Flexner Report was published, but we need not assume that the use of complex terminology is invariably a good thing. However knowledgeable medical students or young physicians may be about fine points of anatomy, complex biochemical reactions and detailed pathophysiology, they are not going to be of much help to patients if they lack an appreciation for the proper approach to medical problems — not itself contingent on a hefty medical vocabulary. As we've seen, medical students in North America are given much more credit for learning trivia than for learning to do a proper physical examination. This, for instance, presents a contrast with British medical students who (judging from the ones I have met) appear to be more oriented towards the acquisition of practical knowledge and skills.

Medical terminology does, of course, facilitate communication among physicians in many (though by no means all) situations. On the other hand, medical vocabulary can lessen a physician's ability to communicate with lay people. I was confronted with this in my third year. To help finance my education, I wrote an occasional article for the university's alumni journal. On one occasion the editor asked me to do a piece on research in the university. Prior to my entry into medical school, I had written a similar article on medical research, which had been well received; I looked forward to doing an even better job in the medical section of my article this time, with three years' increased comprehension of the subject. I was certainly taken by surprise, then, when the editor telephoned me for clarification of certain parts of the article. He said I had couched it in excessively complex medical jargon, suggesting that because of my medical studies I had become less sensitive to the average reader's level of comprehension. This was a considerable blow to my ego, since I had taken special pains to write in an easily-understandable way.

This sort of problem also arises when physicians interview patients in the ordinary course of medical practice. Studies of these lopsided dialogues have shown them to be so laden with medical jargon that patients have great difficulties understanding what the physicians say. Barabara Korsch and others at the University of Southern California have examined communication in a pediatrics outpatient department:

An outstanding barrier to communication encountered in more than half the recorded cases is the pediatrician's use of difficult technical language. One mother said on interview that the doctor talked "medical", another mother during an interaction requested that the pediatrician repeat what he had said in "English". The technical terms used apply to the anatomic processes of the child (i.e. nares, labia, sphincter), to physiologic processes (e.g. injection, edema, peristalsis, and so forth), often to laboratory procedures (e.g. lumbar puncture, Coomb's titre, Tine test), and to many other subjects dealt with in medical consultation.[1]

This study and others like it conclude that gaps in communication are greatest when patients are from one of the lower socio-economic groups. The problem of patient comprehension is not limited to highly technical jargon. The misunderstanding of quite basic terms is commonplace. C.M. Boyle has shown that less than twenty per cent of patients can correctly identify the approximate location of the stomach, less than fifty per cent know where the liver is situated and less than sixty per cent know the whereabouts of the urinary bladder.[2]

Many factors contribute to poor communication between physicians and their patients. For one thing, physicians tend to come from socio-economic, educational and cultural backgrounds that make them more likely than many of their patients to regard certain words and phrases as part of the vernacular even before they get to medical school. Besides that, many physicians forget (as I did) how much medical jargon they did not understand before they began their studies, and so without realizing it, use words not comprehended by others.

Furthermore, patients differ, largely according to class, when confronted with patter that they do not understand. More articulate patients will actively seek and usually obtain a satisfactory explanation. Persons who are less articulate, or who tend more to non-verbal means of expression, will receive short shrift because physicians are less sensitive to these forms of communication.

Finally, there are situations in which physicians deliberately use the medical lexicon as a rather heavy-handed tool for maintaining dominance. By making situations incomprehensible to their patients, they can dull the patients' critical abilities and impose their own preference for a particular therapeutic option.

This all adds up to one further element in the stratification of the relationship between physicians and patients: the jargon that doctors use relegates patients to a relatively passive role in therapy. But is the medical jargon really essential in all situations?

In fact, almost anything physicians have to say (not merely those things they have to say to patients) could be said in a way that *almost any* person could understand. To communicate in this way would probably mean that physicians would have to increase the amount of time spent with their patients, but not by all that much. That physicians do not speak "English" reflects the social structure of medical practice, for it is not only their patient-clients who are left out in the cold by the jargon. Other health workers are excluded from meaningful participation in rounds, conferences and even one-to-one encounters because they cannot "speak the jive". Those who cannot dare not impose their opinions on others who are so much more "knowledgeable".

It would be inappropriate, however, to condemn the use of technical medical terms in all instances and, undeniably, there are occasions when efficiency is enhanced by shop-talk. It would not improve the practice of medicine, for example, if physicians had to explain to their colleagues the phenomenon of obstruction of a coronary artery by a blood clot and the subsequent damage to the heart muscle caused by loss of blood supply, when the term **myocardial infarction** conveys the same information much more concisely. That does *not* mean that they couldn't give a fairly detailed explanation of the same thing in simple language to a patient with coronary artery disease. Their failure to communicate in this way leads most other health workers and patients to accept the physisician's primacy.

Not all do. As Barbara Korsch indicates, many rebel openly against such subjugation.[3] But many more accept their passive role in therapy unquestioningly and even willingly. According to Korsch, the use of complex medical jargon is associated with a high rate of patient satisfaction. Many consider it a compliment to their intelligence to be spoken to in such technical (even if incomprehensible) jargon![4] This is quite consistent with the concept of the sick role, which allows people to escape from their normal obligations into a situation where they are subject to the physician's authority. Similarly, the extent to which physicians seek to introduce complex terminology into interviews with patients will match their own inclinations to exercise power over others. If physicians were not seeking to play certain roles in relation to their patients, and if they were more sensitive to the patients' needs, medical jargon would not be a hindrance to effective communication. As it is, the technical language of medicine is one more convenient tool for the establishment of certain dynamics in medical relationships.

Talking about patients

It is not uncommon for a group of physicians, when talking among themselves in the presence of a patient, to use a word or expression they would not normally employ. Their purpose is to ensure that the patient does not grasp the tenor of the conversation.

Sometimes this is done out of consideration. During ward rounds, for example, a house officer might refer to a person's **mitotic lesion** of the lung, something that would be called cancer or carcinoma anywhere but at the bedside. It would be unnecessarily cruel to confront a patient with such an unpleasant reality every time the problem was discussed in his or her presence. Unfortunately, some physicians talk this way when they haven't even informed the patient about the condition; talking about mitotic lesions ritualizes this avoidance of responsibility.

Another expression used to conceal what is being discussed from patients is much more malevolent. From time to time on ward rounds, physicians can be heard to remark to their colleagues that a particular patient has a **supratentorial lesion**. The "lesion" to which they refer is located above the *tentorium cerebelli*, the membrane separating the cerebral hemispheres of the brain above from the cerebellum below. The implication is that the person's symptoms are in the head and, in fact, represent psychosomatic illness. The expression is most often used on a surgical ward in the presence of the patient but not infrequently elsewhere as well. There is not much chance the patient will know what it means; it acts as a kind of behind-the-back insult. Furthermore, saying "this neurotic sonofabitch is wasting my time with imaginary complaints" — as the expression implies — suggests that the physician lacks empathy for the patient and for the very real nature of psychosomatic illness.* This expression says as much about the physician's attitudes as it does about any desire to withhold information from the patient.

There are other expressions used to describe patients, expressions which are never used in their presence for reasons that will become obvious:

Crock: This is a term applied to persons whose complaints are not "organic" (that is, those with supratentorial lesions), and to some who have chronic diseases about which nothing or very little can be done. It is not a complimentary term. Nor is the care of the person to whom it is applied given a high priority by the physician who uses it. Some physicians prefer to talk of **turkeys** or **gomers** rather than crocks.[5]

Piss poor protoplasm: This term, not particularly malicious, is used to describe patients who have disease or failure of several organs or organ systems. It is often used jokingly when a person is succumbing to disease on several fronts. It seems to indicate a regard for the patient as something less than a thinking and feeling human being.

This patient has two neurons: Neurons are nerve cells, and this insulting remark is a house officer's assessment of a patient's intelligence. It is often applied to a patient who is unco-operative in diagnosis or therapy. The physician's dubious logic leads to the conclusion that the failure of the patient to do as told can only be a result of meagre intelligence.

Other terms that physicians use to describe their patients are less derogatory, but even referring to patients on the ward as "good teaching material", or to a person with a rare or complex problem as "an interesting case", tends to negate the image of the physician as a caring person with a concern for humanity.

The roles of the physician

The physician as orthodox moralist: Some medical jargon reflects the particular prejudices or hang-ups of physicians. In any proper medical record, at least some of the important "negatives" will be listed: no cough, no diarrhea, no chest pain, and so on. The work of Korsch and others (cited earlier in this chapter) suggests that at least some of the information physicians collect in their interviews with patients and usually accept on faith, is inaccurate. Ironically, it is only for particular parts of a medical history that many physicians reserve their scepticism, and written medical records reflect this bias: "This patient **denies** sexual contact"; "the patient **claims** he drinks two or three beers a day".

The physician as activist: The authoritarian nature of many interactions between physicians and patients finds expression in a number of terms which reflect the active role of doctors and the passivity of patients. The ministrations of physicians to the ill are frequently called **patient management.** Physicians manage patients and their problems; the patients have little to do but lie back and put up with it.

Accurately or otherwise, physicians take credit for much of what happens to the people under their care. A person who follows a treatment prescribed by a physician, and whose condition subsequently improves, has been **cured by** the physician. A person who visits a physician regularly because of a particular medical problem is being **treated by** the physician, even when no therapy is instituted (on such occasions, the physician's contribution is to manage the patient **conservatively**).

When a physician administers medicine to a patient who is on the brink of death, and who subsequently recovers, the physician will sometimes see this as having **saved a life**, no matter how routine or uncomplicated the treatment has been. When such efforts to save a dying person are attenuated, extensive or unlikely to succeed, they are called **heroics**, although the patient is clearly the one who is enduring. The physician-hero has little more to do than select therapy. So completely does the physician expropriate the active role in therapy that, when a person dies, the physician most often refers to the event as having **lost a patient.***

Physician dominance in relationships with patients is widely acknowledged and rarely questioned, but it is possible for therapeutic activity to be less physician-centred than it is. Only rarely are persons so ill that they are unable to receive recommendations and make their own considered decisions. Rather than identifying physicians as the ones who lose a patient or save a life, they might more properly be looked upon as the ones who play a role (usually relatively small) in an event that most profoundly affects the person to whom it is happening.

The physician as boss: There is one phrase that attests to the dominance of physicians over patients and other health workers as well: **Doctor's Orders**. This phrase, used to describe a physician's recommendations to a patient, implies that the patient has no choice but to do whatever told. The place of Doctor's Orders among health workers is manifested by the presence on every ward of **order sheets** and **order books**. Physicians write down orders for nursing care, diagnostic procedures and therapy. This is rarely done in consultation with nurses or other health workers. I have often seen the night nurse-on-duty wince as she studied the orders some physician had written relating to a new patient, calculating in her mind what it will add up to in the way of work.

Physicians are often insensitive to the impact of their orders on the work of nurses and other people. I have worked on some wards where the head nurses held weekly conferences principally devoted to determining whether or not patients who were having their vital signs checked every two, three or four hours really needed to have them done so often; the house officers tended to forget to discontinue orders for frequent examinations when they ceased to be necessary.

The dominance of physicians is also exemplified by the use of the word **armamentarium** to describe the tools used to diagnose and fight disease: are they not great military strategists masterminding the movements of their footsoldiers in the battle against the Enemy?

The physician as potent: Some idioms denote physicians' belief in their own potency. When patients are to be given medication, this is sometimes expressed as **hitting** them with it; if the medication is given by intravenous infusion, it is called an **I.V. push**. Occasionally, the administering of a large dose of a medication is referred to as **zapping** the patient, but zapping more usually describes the use of electric countershock in the effort to resuscitate a person who has had a cardiac arrest. Finally, when physicians write **stat** next to an order, it means that it is to be done immediately.

The physician as omniscient: The use of some terms denies any limit to physicians' knowledge, by obscuring the fact that doctors do not know the cause of some diseases. When hypertension is of un-known cause (the vast majority of cases), it is called **essential** hyper-tension. Similarly, when the source of an infection or inflammation is not apparent, the disease process is described as **idiopathic**. When a tumour is of a type that makes it difficult to say from what organ or cell line it originated, it is called **undifferentiated.** These words are not for hiding doctors' ignorance from patients (in whose presence they are rarely used), but I would suggest that they help to make the uncertainty of a situation less apparent to physicians themselves.

The physician as infallible: Sometimes patients can become ill because of therapy administered by physicians. (This can happen even when the therapy chosen is appropriate to the circumstances.) When this occurs, physicians never say that the illness is physician-induced. Instead they slip into the more comfortable Greek formulation: the disease is **iatrogenic** (from *Iatros,* physician).

The expressions used to denote a patient's death, or the fact that a patient is dying, obscure that important fact and thereby reinforce the notion of the physician's infallibility. A person who is dying is often said to have a condition that is **terminal.** In some hospitals, a patient near death is said to be **skating down the tube.** When death comes, a patient doesn't die but **expires**, or **arrests** (or does nothing at all while the physician **loses the patient**). A dead person who arrives that way at the Emergency Room is a **D.O.A.** (dead on arrival). At one large American medical centre, the person who dies on a hospital ward is called a **Brady** (for the Brady pavilion where the pathology department is located.)

When I was a first year medical student, I witnessed the death of an elderly woman, and the unsuccessful attempt at resuscitating her. While resuscitation efforts were still under way (but when it had begun to appear that they were not going to succeed), the physician I was with commented: "It will be interesting to see what the pathologist has to say about this case."

I was puzzled. If the pathologist was going to have a say, did that mean that this person was dead or about to die? If so, why not say so? Since then, I have heard this same expression repeated many times. Most recently it occured when a woman was seriously ill with an unknown malady that seemed likely to kill her. The woman walked out of the hospital perfectly well, but not before an intern had expressed interest in what the pathologist was going to say about her. Clearly this is a convenient way for physicians to avoid the reality that there is nothing they can do for a particular person.

Abbreviations

D.O.A. is not the only abbreviation that has attained popular acceptance in medical communication; the jargon is full of such expressions, and they take some getting used to.

The first time I heard a classmate refer to the hematocrit* as **the 'crit**, and to the electrolytes* as **the 'lytes**, I had to restrain my laughter, but I soon discovered that he had learned earlier than many of us to emulate our physician-teachers in referring to laboratory tests by their abridged names. In some instances, the use of abbreviated names to describe laboratory tests simplifies discussion. Who wants to say 'serum glutamic oxaloacetate transaminase' when **SGOT** will do just as well? Similarly, **T3** is less of a mouthful than is 'triiodothyronine'.

On the other hand, it is not much simpler to say **P.R.A.** than 'plasma renin activity'. This particular test is a new one, strongly advocated by some doctors as useful in the screening of hypertensive patients; it helps determine which ones should be admitted to hospital for further investigation. The use of the test means that many people will be hospitalized before they are treated for their hypertension, even though it is far from clear that the in-hospital investigation makes any difference to the treatment they will receive.* Nevertheless, giving this dubious test an abbreviated name confers upon it a legitimacy it might not otherwise possess. Referred to in this way, it appears to be part of the physician's "armamentarium", which probably helps it to gain acceptance in the medical community.

Abbreviations are also commonly used in the description of symptoms, diseases and body parts. They are intended to make communication more efficient, but their use inevitably makes it more difficult for those not familiar with the expressions to follow and participate in discussions. One physician who came to work in Montreal after studying medicine in France was assigned to a cardiology ward when he first arrived in the hospital. One expression he kept running into was **M.I.**, the abbreviation for myocardial infarction or heart attack. Everyone in cardiology talks about M.I.s, day and night. Not knowing what an M.I. was and being ashamed to ask, naturally it was a matter of some embarrassment to him. But all medical students have similar experiences of being accosted with an abbreviation that, it would seem, they are supposed to know, but do not. The first time a classmate told me about a patient with **C.B. and E** (chronic bronchitis and emphysema), I didn't have a clue what he was talking about, having only heard that disorder described as **COLD** (chronic obstructive lung disease) or **COPD** (chronic obstructive pulmonary disease). Fortunately, I had the courage to admit my ignorance and ask him what the hell he meant.

It is not unusual, but quite confusing, to come across more than one abbreviation for the same thing. Shortness of breath on exertion — **SOBOE** — is also called **DOE** — dyspnea on exertion. The functional inquiry into a patient's history of symptoms and illnesses is abbreviated in the medical record as either the **FI** or the **ROS** (review of systems).*

Finally, medical records abound with abbreviations. Some adept house officers can do most of a workup on a patient without using one complete word. However, when someone writes **HEENT-NAD**, which means "head, ears, eyes, nose, throat — no abnormality discovered", it is a pretty safe bet that the physician has not bothered to examine this part of the patient's body very carefully.* By writing the results of their work up in this abbreviated form, physicians are able to ritualize and perhaps abbreviate an examination they know is supposed to be complete.

Cardiac arrest

There is one group of expressions that allows the discussion of a ticklish subject within earshot of patients without upsetting them, and each hospital uses one expression from the group. **Ninety-nine. Code blue. Two-three.** When one of these phrases booms out over a hospital's public address system, everyone who works there knows that a cardiac arrest has occured and an attempt at resuscitation is to be made. "Two-three on eight medical. Two-three on eight medical." The members of the cardiac arrest team leave whatever they are doing and run to the eighth floor of the medical wing, where they will attempt to correct, using electric countershock and medications, the irregular rhythm of a person's heart, which will otherwise be fatal. When a two-three (or a ninety-nine) is announced, few if any patients know what is going on, and their burden of stress is thus minimized.

If the cardiac arrest code word were only used in the situation of a cardiac arrest, its use would be beyond reproach. However, it is also used in discussions about patients who *might* die, which is quite another thing. When a person is admitted to the hospital, there is always the possibility, however remote, that he or she will not leave the place alive. It is routine procedure for the cardiac arrest team to be called when a patient dies suddenly. For some patients, however, a decision is taken beforehand *not* to attempt resuscitation in the case of sudden death. This decision is sometimes, but not always, taken in consultation with the relatives of the ill person.*

The decision not to resuscitate is frequently made in the case of a person dying of cancer or some other irreversible disease, someone who seems to have reached the end of the road in spite of all treatment. In such cases, the physician's unilateral decision is at least understandable.

In other cases the decision is not so clear-cut: for instance, when a patient is old, debilitated and (in the judgement of the physician) has "nothing left to live for".* When the decision not to attempt resuscitation has been made, a note is written in the nurse's cardex to that effect. Since this act is rarely acknowledged (and slightly illegal), the **no two-three** is written in pencil so that it can later be erased. In one hospital, the system is even more sophisticated. The head nurse on each ward inserts a square of green cardboard into the cardex, over the card belonging to each doomed patient; this allows the nurse-on-duty to know at a glance whether anything is to be done if a patient's heart stops beating.

A physician usually informs the nurse orally of the decision to let a patient die. One resident showed me a rather clever way of putting this message down on paper. He used to write: "If the patient's condition deteriorates, the physician and family should be notified," meaning that if the patient dies the cardiac arrest team should not be called; instead, those concerned should be informed.

There are other ways in which the two-three business can and does get abused. I recall several conversations about the sorry plight of a patient during which someone asked: "Is he a two-three?" In the context, the distasteful implication of this query was: "Is this pitiful person's life worth an attempted resusitation?"

It is not only the house staff that looks at a patient through glasses tinted with the resusitation status. From orderlies to attending physicians, everyone tempers their relations with and attitudes toward a person in hospital with the knowledge of what is to be done if that person's heart stops. Physicians regularly spend less time with such patients. Everyone avoids getting too involved with them.* To some extent, this represents a difficulty in dealing with dying people on the part of the hospital staff. Giving a special designation to such people spells out for everyone who they are and how they should be treated.

Epinyms

The language of medicine would be at least somewhat less complex if it were not for the widespread use of epinyms. Epinyms are the surnames of physicians, pathologists, physiologists and others, which have come to be attached to a variety of medical phenomena.

The lucky person is usually the one who first publishes a description of the disease or phenomenon. Thus the clinical signs that suggest the diagnosis of infection of the valves of the heart are designated **Osler's nodes, Roth spots** and **Janeway's nodes.***

The phenomena represented by these epinyms might be more easily remembered if the "proper" Latin and Greek names were used. (I always had trouble remembering which nodes were Osler's and which belonged to Janeway.) There are really only two reasons for using epinyms. Firstly, physicians love to name things after themselves. Secondly, a physician able to drop epinyms into a conversation appears to be extremely erudite, particularly when the epinyms used are applied to obscure phenomena. But this "erudition" makes it much more difficult for people unfamiliar with the terminology to participate meaningfully in medical discussions.

A jargon for each specialty

The physicians who practise in each specialty have their own subcategories of medical jargon, with expressions that either convey information specific to their disciplines or reflect their own particular attitudes. For instance, much of what internists say is incomprehensible to other specialists; they use epinyms more than any other doctors. Surgeons have the gruffest shop-talk of all: operations are called **going in, cutting** or **splitting the belly.** Quite aside from the Freudian implications, such phrases probably contribute to the depersonalization of care.

Surgeons are also the foremost users of expressions such as "interesting case" and "good pathology". You sometimes hear them using another expression, one that invokes a perspective they share with no other group of physicians: "When in doubt, cut it out."

Psychiatrists have a jargon of their own, of course, but they do have one word that probably represents them better than any other: **schizophrenia.** The diagnosis of schizophrenia, it seems, is affixed by psychiatrists on their patients with alarming eagerness and the diagnosis, once made, preordains the nature of the relationship. "Three-quarters of the people on this ward are schizophrenics," I was told when I first set foot on a psychiatric ward; I don't think this sort of attitude was an encouragement to come to an understanding of such people and of the nature of their problems.

Pediatricians have a less abrasive jargon, most probably because of the unique nature of their patients. A children's hospital is often affectionately referred to as **The Kids.*** When pediatricians talk about newborns (and some not-so-tiny patients as well), they often say **it,** meaning the child. It is understandable that they think of some of their patients as neuter: some are so small and so sick that it is hard to see them as anything more than a collection of desperately serious problems. And a child with an unusual appearance invariably arouses excitement on a pediatrics ward; often there is some rare genetic disorder involved. The pediatrics staff might call such a child a **funny face** or an **F.L.K.** (funny-looking kid).

Pediatrics hospitals are also more receptive to visitors than general hospitals are; the staff expects the child's mother to be around quite a bit of the time and affectionately refer to her as **Mom**. Similarly, pediatrics workers are less callous about patients with fatal or incurable disorders. Sensing, perhaps, the magnitude of the tragedy of a little child being deathly ill, people go to great lengths to act humanely towards them and their kin. In fact, pediatricians and other pediatrics workers are often the most considerate and least authoritarian people in the hospital. This may be a result of the patients they are dealing with: children tend to be less predictable than adults and rarely are willing to conform to hospital rules; they might cry during physical examinations or run up and down the corridors, trying to be themselves. These are signs of health on a pediatrics ward; a patient who behaves this way elsewhere in a hospital is labelled **unco-operative.***

Prescription drugs

No discussion of the jargon of medicine would be complete without something being said about that greatest source of new medical words, the pharmaceutical industry. The drug manufacturers have graciously supplied us with tens of thousands of words, the names of the products they sell.

When a new drug is marketed, it is identified by three names. First, there is the **chemical name**, which typically is painfully long, contains several syllables, and is punctuated with numbers and hyphens. This name is usually hard to say and impossible to remember, so with government approval the company developing the product also assigns a simpler **generic** name. This generic name thereafter appears on every company's brand of that particular product.

In addition all of the large corporations that produce a particular medication assign a third name to it, their **brand name**. It is this last name that pharmaceutical manufacturers attempt to impress, through advertising, upon the hearts and minds of physicians. Despite the fact that, with rare exceptions, there is no demonstrable benefit to patients of having one brand prescribed rather than another, these companies spend several thousand dollars per physician per year "educating" them about the superiority of their products over those of their competitors.

The company that introduces a pill or medication has a patent on it for several years. During this time, it is important for the company to impress the name of its product on the physicians (who control consumption), to convince them that it is not only preferable to other types of medication used to treat the same condition, but also the only legitimate embodiment of the (generic) medication. This second objective is important because, when the patent expires, a free-for-all generally ensues, in which the originating company's price is usually undercut by competitors. *

Since the companies that patent the products are also able to choose their generic names, it is not surprising that they assign such forgettables as **iodochlorhydroxyquin**, so that physicians will remember the products by their brand names instead. * Generic names are consistently and considerably longer than brand names.[6]

Brand names of pills (like those of any other marketed goods) are not chosen haphazardly. Those medications intended to kill pain, to calm nerves and to lower blood pressure have soft, soothing names (which are also, at least occasionally, sexually suggestive to those uttering them): **Valium, Darvon, Hydrodiuril, Inderal, Serpasil, Dyrenium, Librium.** "Big Job" medications have harsher names: **Keflin** (an antibiotic recommended for use in certain serious infections), **Hyperstat** (for reducing blood pressure in an emergency), **Cytoxan** (used in the treatment of some cancers).*

The marketing people do their jobs well: give-aways to physicians of medical equipment, calendars, free dinners; free trips to "conferences" on their products; advertisements; detail men coming around with free samples (and advice), and so on. Many physicians do not even know offhand the generic names of the medications they prescribe.* Some names become so institutionalized that it is actually inappropriate to use their generic equivalents in conversation (although reputable medical journals use only the generic names).

Lasix is such a product. It is a brand name for **furosemide,** a medicine which removes salt and water from the body. It is useful to administer furosemide in an emergency to a person with acute congestive heart failure, who needs to have some fluid removed rapidly. At least a few times daily in every Emergency Room, someone can be heard saying: "Give the patient forty [milligrams] of **Lasix.**" It is rare that anyone asks for "furosemide" in an emergency: the name doesn't ring true in the same way. **Lasix** is as much a part of medical jargon as the parts of the body and the

names of diseases. Not surprisingly, the universal familiarity with
its name has helped to promote its use in non-emergency situations
when much less expensive drugs would do just as well. A second
brand of furosemide recently became available in Canada, but without a name like **Lasix** it probably will have trouble making an impression on the market.

There are other ways in which brand names can become institutionalized. Some physicians administer furosemide in a test
that is supposed to distinguish different types of hypertension. This
has become known as the 'Lasix test'. Another test, sometimes performed on people with myasthenia gravis (a disorder of the junc-
tions between nerves and the muscles they supply), involves the
administration of a drug called **edrephonium;** the test is called, after
the brand name of the medication, the 'Tensalon test'.

When a certain tranquilizer, which is now one of the bestselling prescription drugs, was first being marketed some years ago,
it was distributed free for use within hospitals. Physicians accustomed themselves to prescribing it within the hospital and, of
course, carried this habit out into their offices. Now there are other
brands of this medication, but none can touch it for sales.

There are many more subtleties to the game of selecting a name
for a medication and marketing it. One physician told me, for example, that he prescribes the brand of penicillin called **P-50**, only because it takes less time to write. Neither he nor I knew how its price
compared to that of any other brand; it was a source of some embarrassment to him when we looked it up and discovered that it was
one of the most expensive brands of **benzyl penicillin** on the market.

The medical school course on medications and their uses
(pharmacology and therapeutics) is oriented to the use of generic
names.* There are rare exceptions to a general rule that might be
stated as "All aspirin are pretty much alike." Nevertheless, medical
students do pick up the brand name habit (usually on hospital wards)
and once they do it is hard for them to kick it. The use of generic
names is looked upon with disfavour by many people who work in
hospitals and who are accustomed to brand names. Once, working
in the Emergency Room, I asked a nurse to give five milligrams of
diazepam (generic name) to a patient who was having a seizure.
"Around here, we call it Valium, and that's what you damn well are
going to call it if you want your patient to get any," she retorted.

The extent to which the effective marketing of brand names can
overwhelm even the most critical individuals was impressed upon
me during a pharmacology lecture in my third year. A lecturer was

talking about how important it was for us not to be conned into the use of brand names on the prescriptions we would write as physicians. As he was making a particular point about **reserpine** (used to treat hypertension), he inadvertently said **Serpasil** (the brand name) instead. Class members rolled in the aisles with laughter, but it was really not very funny.

The mystification of patients is also part of the drug name game. The names of many medications are not written on the prescription bottle, and even when they are, patients are often not told what they are for. This can lead to that frequently recurring scene in the Emergency Room in which a physician desperately needs to know the name of a medication the patient has been taking but all the patient is able to say is "the little white pills". In other situations, patients will know the brand name of a medication, expecting that their doctors will know it too. It may be a bitter pill for physicians to swallow if they are obliged to admit that they do not know this one of thousands of brand names on the market.

It is impossible for physicians to master all the brand names; this should encourage them to think generically, but they do not, clinging instead to the more familiar brand names. As one drug advertisement reassures them: "There are twenty-five brands of **chlordiazepoxide** in Canada, but only one **Librium**."

One fellow I interned with sought to demystify the racket. He substituted the expression **proper name** for generic name and, instead of brand name, he spoke of **advertising name,** making it clear just what were the issues involved. Unfortunately, he was in a minority.

Is there a pattern to the different uses of medical jargon I have surveyed in this chapter? The jargon physicians use reflects and reinforces certain realities while obscuring others. Because we live in an era that has seen rapid expansion in science and technology, there is a great deal of technical jargon. Because we live in a society in which private enterprises can produce new kinds of medications almost at will, there are many thousands of new products on the market, all with different names. Because physicians maintain a dominant position in their relationships to other health workers and to patients, other words that reflect these relationships make their way into the lexicon. Because physicians are not related to others through their work in the most humane of ways (and this problem is certainly not limited to medical practice) they are sometimes unable to confront situations — such as death and dying — without invoking jargon that will obscure the reality at hand. Other doctor talk expresses the inhumane, or even antagonistic, attitudes of physicians to some of their patients.

The jargon being used might be the epinym for a disease, the abbreviation for a symptom, an insult to the patient or a euphemism for dying. But medical shop talk is not responsible for the social and occupational stratification of the hospital, the dynamics of the physician-patient relationship and the attitudes of physicians. Language use is also a function of the complex interaction between technological evolution, the political and economic organization of society and the social relations among that society's members. This is no less true in medicine than anywhere else in society.

Notes

page 168: Sometimes patients whose illnesses — while not necessarily psychosomatic — are of uncertain origin, are also said to have supratentorial lesions.

page 169: In fact, the very word "patient" carries with it an implication of passivity. Besides the more familiar usage, *The Oxford English Dictionary* lists the following definitions:
3. A person subjected to the supervision, care, treatment, or correction of someone.
4. A person or thing that undergoes some action, or to whom or which something is done...
The dictionary quotes John Wesley as saying: "He that is not free is not an Agent but a Patient."

page 172a: The percentage of the blood's volume consisting of red blood cells.

172b: The sodium, potassium and chloride concentrations in the blood serum.

172c: Some medical journals have commented upon this problem editorially. (See "When to measure renin", *Lancet* [editorial] 1 [1975]: 783-784.)

page 173a: In one of my earliest clinical experiences, I was admonished for writing "ROS" instead of "FI" in a case history.

173b: One resident used to say that "NAD" really means 'no assessment done'!

173c: Advice may be sought directly or indirectly from relatives about possible resuscitation. Often a physician just looks for some hint that the relatives of a person who is dying would not be too upset if the patient were allowed to "go" peacefully. When such hints are not forthcoming, physicians must either put the question bluntly to families (which is hard to do), or decide on their own.

page 174a: I leave it to the reader to speculate on the biases that can creep into such a decision-making process. When that octogenarian humanist Francisco Franco was obviously dying (or even dead), no one thought it necessary to cease "heroic" measures to save his life. The same week, I was called to the bedside of a younger man who had succumbed to a heart attack. As we began resuscitative efforts, an intern scurried in to inform us that this man was in the hospital mainly because he had no place to live, so we needn't be too vigorous in our efforts to save his life.

174b: "Not to be resuscitated" is, in some ways, comparable to the designation "unclean".

page 175a: Some other examples: **Crohn's Disease** is an inflammatory disorder of the bowel; the **suspensory ligaments of Cooper** keep the female breast from sagging; **Pott's Disease** is tuberculosis of the spine.

175b: In Toronto, they call it **The Sick Kids'**.

page 176: Of course, pediatrics does have its share of inhumane practitioners, and humanity is regularly absent from pediatrics emergency rooms and outpatient departments. I once asked a middle-aged pediatrician why this was, and he said, "The patients in the emergency room and the clinics come from the slums and the physicians come from the suburbs."

page 177a: Only occasionally have the pharmaceutical corporations been caught fixing prices. But because the "generic" companies (which do sell their products at lower prices) are unable to advertise, they are effectively shut out of the market. This leaves the vast majority of consumers with very well-marketed and very overpriced medications.

177b: That one, incidentally, is marketed as *Vioform*. Likewise, *chlordiazepocide* is better known as *Librium*.

177c: That every anti-cancer regimen has a "dynamic anti-cancer ring" has been the subject of satire in recent medical literature. (See R. McMillan, R.L. Longmire, "Crisis in oncology — acute vowel obstruction [with apologies to oncologists everywhere]", *New England Journal of Medicine* 294 [1978]: 1288-1289.)

177d: Well over 80 percent of prescriptions contain only a brand name.

page 178: Brand names are rarely mentioned, since few pharmacologists take seriously the claims that one brand of a medication is any better than another.

8

Alienation and Authoritarianism in Medicine

Some Conclusions

The method of negation, the denunciation of everything that mutilates mankind and impedes its free development, rests on confidence in man.[1]
—Max Horkheimer

Time and again in this book two concepts have been used to help provide insight into the state of medical education and practice: alienation and authoritarianism. While there are undoubtedly as many ways to study this book's subject as there are writers willing to tackle it, I believe these two concepts provide the most useful framework for focusing on the underlying problems and for interpreting the human interactions observed. The critical social analysis that results from such an approach emphasizes the importance of understanding the relevance to problems in medicine — and elsewhere — of the highly integrated social and economic order in which medicine exists.

Alienation in medicine can only properly be understood in the context of society as a whole. In the modern capitalist world all people who relate to one another in a medical context experience social and productive relations that can generally be described as "alienated". This alienation permeates the activity people undertake in relation to medicine, itself an important part of productive activity today, and in which increasing numbers of people work and hence objectify their labour.* A study of medicine enables the interactions of members of various strata of society to be observed in a common setting: people of different social and economic classes, existing in different relationships to the means of production, coming together either as health workers or as patients.[2] In addition, an understanding of alienation in medicine, and of medicine's role in production, is particularly important at this time when significant elements of human social experience (birth, death, disease, emotional stress) have come to be structured around medical practice, far more than ever before.[3]*

Similarly, authoritarian behaviour, as we've seen, can be observed at most stages of medical education and in almost all areas of hospital medical practice. It too is rooted in a social order that, in various ways, creates much of the need for authoritarianism and encourages its expression.

In earlier chapters we've seen signs of this alienation and authoritarianism as they affect the relationships of medical students to each other, to their pattern of learning and ultimately as doctors to their patients and other health workers as well as to the institutions in which they work. I do not provide solutions to the problems raised in this book — for there are no easy answers — but in this concluding chapter I take a closer look at the concepts mentioned above and attempt to draw some tentative conclusions about their applicability to medicine.

Medicine and alienation
The Marxist theory of alienation

The term "alienation" has been used to convey many different sorts of ideas by philosophers from Grotius to Rousseau to Jean-Paul Sartre.[4] Here we are concerned with only one usage — that derived from the work of Karl Marx. Bertell Ollman has described this as "the intellectual construct in which Marx displays the devastating effect of capitalist production on human beings, on their physical and mental states and on the social processes of which they are a part".[5]

Marx contends that the social relations of every society form a whole, and that the key to the understanding of social, political and other relationships lies in the analysis of their economic underpinnings. In *A Contribution to the Critique of Political Economy* he says, "it is not men's consciousness that determines their existence, but their social existence that determines their consciousness."[6]

In the modern era, much productive activity is strikingly different from that described by Marx. This does not detract from his formulation of the concept of alienation; it merely obliges us to express it in terms of twentieth century conditions and situations, in which alienated capitalist production nevertheless remains the underlying problem.*

For Marx, alienation is not an abstract concept. It is a specific feature of human relationships in a capitalist era and it can only be understood in relation to its opposite: "unalienation", "lack of alienation" or, perhaps most appropriately, "transcendence of alienation". Unalienated people, Hungarian writer Istvan Meszaros notes in his book *Marx's Theory of Alienation*, would realize their potential and satisfy their needs through their labour in a world that would be an expression of both their needs and their potentials; and they would, through social interaction, grow into new needs and new potentialities.[7] Marx's ideal of unalienation is a person who "as a productive social being... transforms the world around him in a specific way, leaving his mark on it".[8]

Marx divided his discussion of human alienation into four major aspects or categories: the alienation of labour or productive activity; alienation from the product of labour; alienation of people's relationships with others around them; and, finally, alienation of people from their "species life". The first three aspects particularly are closely related phenomena; each nourishes and in some way potentiates each of the others.* And all of these aspects can be seen in medical education and in the practice of medicine. We have seen examples throughout the pages of this book.

People are alienated in other ways: in their relationship to nature, and in their senses (aesthetic alienation). In addition, alienation can be examined in a number of dimensions — economic, psychological, political. All of these are, however, but reflections of and variations upon the four main categories of alienation described by Marx.

In his later writings, Marx used the term less often, but it is evident in many of these works that alienation was an important point of reference for an analysis in which he used other expressions, such as the fetishism of commodities, to describe the relations of an alienated society. As German theorist Karl Korsch points out, this was not a significant deviation in his thought.*

Alienation of labour or productive activity

In medicine, as we've seen, there is a tremendous stratification of workers, in both the work they do and the amount of remuneration they receive. At one end of the scale are the doctors, among the highest-paid workers in society. At the other end are workers like the housekeeping and maintenance crews, who are among the lowest-paid.

The people at this lowest-paid level seldom entertain notions that the productive activity in which they engage is anything more than a method of maintaining life. Their work is usually undertaken as a means to acquire money, which in turn satisfies other needs of housing, clothing, food, entertainment and other living expenses. It is external necessities that compel them to play the often demeaning role of a low-ranking health worker. *

"Unskilled" and "semi-skilled" health work is fragmented and specialized; it is very much like assembly-line work that involves responsibility for only an immediate, specified task.[9] There is no place for spontaneity. Any attempt at individual effort would probably be interpreted as a threat to institutional efficiency. (In this kind of setting "efficiency" probably *would* be compromised by any nonconformist efforts; thus is the institutional interest opposed to that of any people who would seek to realize at least some of their potential through their work).

The productive activity of health workers can rarely be an expression of their personalities, humanity and individuality. Their productive activity does not provide them with "new needs and new powers for their gratification".[10] Instead, they may acquire new limitations — accepting the definition of themselves implicit in their work situation, they are inhibited from pursuing other avenues of personal growth. They are required , for instance, to wear uniforms, colour-coded for rank. This is quite consistent with their role in productive activity, which amounts to being machine parts in a health enterprise.

This is an example of what Marx means by the "alienation of labour or productive activity". For these hospital workers, the uniforms, regimentation and abuse by "superiors" merely make explicit what is equally true, if less evident, for other workers: their work is not their life, their expression and realization, their confirmation in the natural world; it is, rather, their alienated productive activity, undertaken of necessity so that, in other ways and at other times they can lead meaningful lives.

It is Marx's view that labour is the one area of activity most significant for human fulfilment and development, because it is through productive activity that people should be able to do those things uniquely human (work towards transforming the world in a way that will leave their own particular mark on it).[11] What, according to Marx, constitutes this alienation of labour?

First, the fact that labour is *external* to the worker, i.e., it does not belong to his essential being; that in his work, therefore, he does not affirm himself but denies himself, does not feel contented but unhappy, does not develop freely his physical and mental energy but mortifies his body and ruins his mind. The worker therefore only feels himself outside his work, and in his work feels outside himself. He is at home when he is not working, and when he is working he is not at home. His labour is therefore not voluntary but coerced; it is *forced labour*. It is not the satisfaction of a need; it is merely a *means* to satisfy needs external to it.[12]

People do not work in order to realize and fulfil themselves in relation to their world: they work in order to survive. They take jobs in which others exploit them, jobs which frequently hold little interest for them beyond the capacity to provide money (which they need to enable them to go about the process of living outside of working hours). The jobs may be expressly designed to require little or no skill; thus workers are easily replaced, expendable. Their work is planned by fiat from above; rarely is there much room for human spontaneity or creativity.* The specialization generally associated with assembly-line production makes labour even more demeaning and exacerbates alienation:

[T]he human qualities and idiosyncracies of the worker appear increasingly as *mere sources of error* . . . Neither objectively nor in relation to his work does man appear as the master of the process; on the contrary, he is a mechanical part incorporated into a mechanical system. He finds it already pre-existing and self sufficient, it functions independently of him and he has to conform to its laws whether he likes it or not.[13]

Employers do not share the workers' perspective. They pay what they consider a fair price to their employees, who have freely entered into the contract to work (although those employees had no real choice). Employers want their workers to be as efficient as possible so they will obtain the maximum return on investment in their labour. Workers have quite different interests, but give up control over their labour when they take a job. *It is the act of taking the job, rather than the conditions of their work, that is responsible for the workers' alienation in their productive activity.*[14]

Productive activity in capitalist society is a force that stands opposed to human nature and its fulfilment. Labour power is a commodity, which a person seeks to exchange for other commodities. As Lukas notes, people become alienated from their productive activity when they contract to sell their labour power in this way.[15]

The middle-level workers in hospitals — the nurses and other professionals — experience somewhat better working conditions than the people at the lowest level of unskilled or semi-skilled work. But they nevertheless endure an oppressive work situation of their own and their productive activity is likewise alienated. Nurses, having sold their labour-power on the marketplace like any commodity, lose the right to direct its use.* As we've seen in earlier chapters, nurses are very restricted in the role they may play in the delivery of health care and often display a mentality of subjugation typical of alienated labour.

Nurses who came into the profession out of idealism rapidly become aware of the limitations placed upon their growth. Those who undertake to become nurses with any but the most limited perspective soon find themselves doing work that betrays their ideals, their aspirations and their conceptions of what their roles should be. Many nurses, in fact, quit work as soon as it is no longer necessary for economic reasons. Others work in order to occupy time that would be otherwise empty or persist in the job out of an inner necessity — the need to do some work, however short its possibilities may fall of the ideal.

But are doctors, those daring and important professionals in the white coats, the subjects of so many television soap operas, also alienated in their work activity? Given their relatively privileged position, it seems unlikely at first glance. However, medicine exists in a specific social context — a society whose organization (and principal mode of production) deprives nearly everyone of the opportunity to partake fully and meaningfully in productive activity.

Physicians have more opportunity than most people to determine the conditions of their labour: they can select any of a number of income levels and types of practice depending on whom they work for and whom they seek to serve. The decisions of most physicians about these matters are based not on internal necessity but on such external contingencies as money, social status and the opportunity to hold power over others in the course of human interaction.

Their businesses would not be as successful as they are if physicians were not conscious of their productive activity being a kind of business. This is not to suggest in any serious way that physicians correspond to the capitalists who own the means of production; they are more like small businessmen. This places them nonetheless in the continuum of production relations in modern society. Physicians who act in their own economic interests are doing what society has conditioned them to do.*

Specialization in medicine (that is, the division of labour) fragments productive activity. Doctors too may feel as though they work on an assembly-line, in spite of their pre-eminent role in the delivery of medical care. Significantly, they may not feel any commitment to — or interest in — the whole process (that is, on a most basic level, the care of the whole patient).*

Isn't the work of the physician fulfilling in at least some respects? What of the physicians who bury themselves in their work to the exclusion of almost all else — "My life is my work"? What other motivation can they have for their incredible devotion to medicine besides the satisfaction they find in their labour?

The work of doctors does have the potential for being less a denial and more an affirmation of life than does the work of an assembly-line worker. Abstractly, there is much to be said for what physicians spend their time doing, and even for the amount of time they spend doing it. In reality, however, their devotion to duty, where it exists, can be motivated by a number of external factors not dependent on an especially fulfilling work situation.

Some physicians work long hours precisely in order to avoid confronting some reality in their lives outside their work. Others do not try to escape their "other lives" in this way and, in fact, find it a considerable hardship to work long hours and be thereby deprived of the opportunity to have real lives outside the hospital. Their long hours are either motivated by a desire for more money or, as in the case of residents and interns, are imposed by hospital bureaucrats.

Those who bury themselves in their work and those who feel trapped in it have much in common. In an unalienated situation, work activity would be integrated with other aspects of a person's existence. Work activity would influence all the person's social interaction and vice versa. The experiences inside and outside of the work setting would be complementary and mutually enriching, an organic whole. This certainly is not the case for most physicians in modern society.*

The alienation of physicians is not comparable in all respects to that of other kinds of workers. Partly because the economic return for their productive activity is much greater, they are less disturbed than most by the limitations their alienated productive activity places on opportunities for fulfilment.*

The difference of perspective between physicians and, say, factory workers, makes it apparent that, although they are both alienated under capitalism, the consequences of the alienation differ. This clearly illustrates the concept of "class consciousness", as defined by George Lukacs:

By relating consciousness to the whole of society it becomes possible to infer the thoughts and feelings which men would have in a particular situation if they were able to assess both it and the interests arising from it in their impact on immediate action and on the whole structure of society. That is to say, it would be possible to infer the thoughts and feelings appropriate to their objective conditions.[16]

Because some people are more comfortable than others in their alienation, Lukas concludes, "*Only the consciousness of the proletariat can point the way that leads out of the impasse of capitalism.*"[17]

Thus, while physicians may be no less alienated than other workers, an understanding of the full devastation of human potential wrought by capitalist production is best achieved through an examination of the condition of the working class. Furthermore, it is through the working class consciousness that the alienation of physicians from their productive activity (and similarly, alienation of other middle-class workers from their productive activity) can be placed in its proper perspective.

Alienation from the product of labour

Since it is through work and what is produced through work that people have a chance to affirm their existence — express their humanity and individuality and fulfil their needs, hopes and potentials — the extent to which the product of this activity fails to permit self-affirmation is also a measure of alienation.* According to Marx:

The worker is related to the product of his labour as to an alien object. The object he produces does not belong to him, dominates him, and only serves in the long run to increase his poverty.... On this premise it is clear that the more the worker spends himself, the more powerful becomes the alien world of objects which he has created over and against himself, the poorer he himself — his inner world — becomes, the less belongs to him as his own. [18]

In the hospital setting, low-ranking health workers have specific duties to perform, duties imposed by others, the results of which are not theirs to mediate. Once the task is completed, the health workers' relation to the product of their labour ceases. Only rarely do they conceive of the product of their labour as belonging to themselves and, even on those rare occasions, no one else shares the delusion; indeed, their contributions pass virtually unnoticed. The product of labour is not in any respect an expression of individuality; its form is preordained according to someone else's will and it is the workers who must adjust to the specifications of the task to be completed, rather than the outcome of the task being their personalized mark upon the world.*

The product of the labour of health workers generates a demand for its use, and hence for more labour. For example, large numbers of technicians operate complex pieces of machinery that add to the prestige of the hospital and provide services sought after by both physicians and patients; but these services do not necessarily improve the ability of the institution to care for the sick. This demand (for the product of their labour) affects health workers no less than anyone else. Yet they have no claim at all on the product of their labour except, as the next consumer, in the market-place of commodities. *

The presumed product of the labour of physicians and nurses is health. Their alienation from this product parallels, in at least some respects, the experience of other health workers.

Because their tasks are so specialized (particularly in the hospital, where medical care is being increasingly concentrated), physicians and nurses rarely have an opportunity to promote health, *per se,* even in theory. They attempt, rather, to promote a small part of health. And their view of how to promote health becomes obscured by self-interest. The maximization of income, an economic interest, can be furthered through unnecessary tests, examinations and even operations (such as the questionable tonsillectomies that many ear, nose and throat specialists continue to perform), and through limitation of membership in the medical profession (which, in Flexnerian tradition, is advanced as being necessary for the maintenance of "professional standards"). Personal self-interest may also be found in the form of self-esteem and loyalty to a point of view propounded by an individual's specialty. These factors may motivate an approach to investigation and treatment of diseases in a way that maximizes use of the specialty's "territory".* Thus, through alienated labour, even idealistic medical practitioners can lose sight of their objective — health.

Health care is profoundly affected by its social context. Practitioners who treat a person with lung disease caused by cigarettes and pollutants have little control over the product of their labour (which in this case could be defined as the amelioration of lung disease), since the disease is a function of the social process and is intimately linked to the needs and the consequences of the mode of production.* The effect specialists have on their product is miniscule compared to these other forces. They can only adjust to the demands the "chronic lunger" makes upon them.*

In addition, patients' compliance with therapy is often poor, a situation brought about largely by social factors. As part of the "medicine machine", however, physicians rarely have much idea of what happens further along the assembly line, and are often not even aware when their patients are avoiding therapy.*

In at least some situations, then, physicians' influence over the product of their endeavours is small and they certainly do not make a significant impression upon the world through what they "produce". The product, health, may easily suffer when it conflicts with the economic return on each physician's productive activity. The most frequent example is the decison made by physicians about how much time to spend with each patient. At least up to a point, the quality of service rendered is proportional to the amount of time devoted to each consultation. Yet when they are being paid on a piece-work basis, the more time they spend with each patient, the fewer consultations completed in the course of the day and the less earned.*

The need felt by physicians-in-training to gain experience in the handling of particular medical situations is also a manifestation of alienation from their product. With competitive training program-mes emphasizing the hurried acquisition of skills, physicians-in-training encounter many situations where they have to choose bet-ween seeking advice before instituting therapy (which could only improve the quality of care) and making a difficult decision on their own (which, besides being good for experience, frequently helps to fulfil another alienated need: to exercise authority over others). Often, the stronger the tendency to try to gain "experience" at an early stage of training, the greater is the cost to the patient's health.*

When medical practice is alienated, medical practitioners often find their "product" to be a separate, opposed and hostile entity, over which there is little or no control. This is similar to Marx's view of alienation from the product of labour:

The alienation of the worker in his product means not only that his labour becomes an object, an *external* existence, but that it exists *outside him*, inde-pendently, as something alien to him, and that it becomes a power on its own confronting him. It means that the life which he has conferred on the object confronts him as something hostile and alien.[19]

As we've seen, physicians become so isolated on the assembly-line of activities meant to produce health that they are not even aware of the conditions necessary for its attainment in the real world (such as the many social factors that influence health and affect the outcome of medical practice on health). Physicians in an unalienated medical practice would make it a matter of priority to master the social as well as the technical contingencies of health, and they would rightly regard this as integral to their own interests.

Alienation of people from one another

The alienation in people's relationships with others around them does not exist in the abstract (as some existentialists would have us believe), nor is it merely an internally-motivated withdrawal from society (one Hegelian formulation). Alienation from one's fellow beings is a consequence of specific social and economic conditions in capitalist societies where "every person speculates on creating a new need in another, so as to drive him to a fresh sacrifice, to place him in a new dependence."[20] What this means is that every person who hopes to prosper economically in capitalist society has to enter into socio-economic relationships that are self-beneficial. That is, people have to seek to establish those relationships that most read-ily allow them to profit from their dealings with others — at the latter's expense.

In medicine this aspect of alienation occurs both in relationships among health workers and in interactions between health workers and patients. As we've seen, inhumane and authoritarian relationships are commonplace. The interpersonal relationships that result are neither healthful expressions of the social individual nor even necessary contingencies of the circumstances in which medicine is practised. Most often, these relationships are expressions of the sadistic and masochistic strivings of individuals looking for escape from the consequences of alienated social relations:

[T]hrough estranged labour . . . man creates the relationship in which other men stand to his production and to his product, and the relation in which he stands to these other men."[21]

In the hospital hierarchy, almost all health workers play stereotypical and predictable roles and the terms of reference for any relationship are woven into the fabric of the uniforms worn. Meaningful human interaction rarely occurs between those whose status differs markedly. Physicians of different status are separated by social barriers almost as often as are health workers with different occupations. The lines of this caste-like differentiation are drawn most explicitly in the cafeteria but are equally true on the wards.

Physicians and other health workers are alienated from their patients in two ways. First, their alienated productive activity, and the alienated product of that activity — as reflected in the economic imperatives dictating the amount of time that can be spent with each patient — hamper positive and humane relationships from being established. Secondly, patients exist in a relationship of dependence to their physicians. Physicians have a monopoly on the product of their labour and this allows them to fulfil their own alienated needs (for example, in the search for potency to exercise authority over patients.)

Alienation from species life

Species life, according to Marx, is all that which differentiates human beings from other animals. A person's alienation from species life is expressed by all that has been given up personally under capitalism, compared to all of which the person is capable. The alienated relationships to productive activity contribute prominently to this for, as Marx says, productive activity is the life of the species. People are alienated from their species life because their lives are not a realization of their potential but an effort to stay alive through their (alienated) labour.

In tearing away from man the object of his production . . . estranged labour tears from him his *species life*, his real objectivity as a member of the species and transforms his advantage over animals into the disadvantage that his organic body, nature, is taken away from him. Similarly, in degrading spontaneous, free, activity, to a means, estranged labour makes man's species life a means to his physical existence.[22]

The species-alienation of health workers, then, is the extent to which the sum of their social and economic relations falls short of the state of being whole, completed beings. The explicit objective of their endeavours (the product, health) is obstructed by a social order that is often antagonistic to it. And their actual work activity falls short of what they are capable of accomplishing. Medical work allows for little human individuality in the execution of the tasks at hand, much less provides workers with an opportunity to transform the world into a place to contemplate, understand and develop themselves. Instead, health workers are transformed by their work into a shell of their former selves. The work lowers their horizons and narrows their potentialities. Even those who recognize that they are unfulfilled lose the sense of their human possibilities.

Productive activity in medicine should have great potential as a form of species life: potential for creatively and resoundingly affirming the workers' sense of being human. Its failure to realize this potential is not merely a failing of the people who do the work. It is principally a consequence of a social order based on alienated production relationships. Even the most idealistic endeavours to heal the sick and prolong life are diminished by alienated society.* Medical teams work hard, for example, to pull their patients through various crises of alcohol-related liver diseases and pollutant-related lung diseases only to send them back, somewhat restored, into the social situation that precipitated their maladies in the first place.

Alienation of the patient

The alienation of the consumer of health services is complex and multidimensional. Patients come to medical care from their own place in productive activity, whether that be in housework, factory work, saleswork or the work of a corporate executive, and in their lives they experience alienation with varying degrees of discomfort. They do not leave that alienated existence behind them when they seek medical services.

Medical care is often sought for reasons springing from alienation. Productive activity is the cause of some disorders (silicosis, work injuries, for instance). Some patients seek medical care because their social relations and species life are alienated and they want to find the apparent escape from an intolerable existence that the "sick role" provides. Others may feel the need to submit to authority, or to palliate a disease whose causation is at least partly social, or to seek institutional help with health problems they should be able to handle on their own.*

Patients are alienated in their relationships to the institutions of medicine, such as hospitals, which are intimidating and confusing, and to medical services, which are rarely designed to maximize patient convenience and accessibility. That these institutions and services are not rationally arrayed according to what is socially most appropriate — the needs of consumers — can be attributed to the bureaucracies that control them, which are subject to the influence of groups seeking to advance their own particular economic or other interests.

The relationship of the patients (who as consumers and taxpayers pay the shot) to their physicians (who fare so well economically) is another feature of patient alienation. Extracting from their labours much more money than most other workers do from theirs, physicians do not even attempt to minimize the impact of the alienated underpinning of medical practice by prescribing the less expensive generic brands of medication. This too is evidence of an alienated relationship between patients and physicians; if the relationship were not alienated, physicians would see their patients' interests as being synonymous with their own. Also, as we've seen earlier, social class has an impact on the service rendered, often hindering effective comunications.

Some important elements of alienation that people experience as patients are related to the general problem of the "fetishism of commodities" — the Marxian concept indicating that under capitalism people have come to look on their social relations with others as relations between objects or commodities.[23]* Medical care and health are not thought of as the products of human endeavour and of the relationships between people; instead, they have been reduced to commodities.* Moreover, the people who provide health services are not regarded as fellow citizens whose labour power just happens to be invested in such activities, and who come to know, as a result, a little more about the function and dysfunction of the body than the patient does. Instead of being treated as consultants, there to help the patients arrive at the best decisions for themselves, doctors are accorded special powers and titles. In these circumstances, patients are likely to lose sight of their own capacities for healing themselves, and can easily overestimate the influence of therapists on the course of their diseases.

The fetishism of commodities means that inanimate objects and institutions are accorded needs, capacities and characteristics that really reflect human activity. One such characteristic of medical care is that it has a price. That it is not a right, easily accessible and comfortably provided to all, is accepted by many who could not imagine it otherwise. For the poor, even when medical care is "free", it often involves long waits for impersonal services in large hospital clinics.* They tolerate this with the feeling that medical care is a product they want badly enough to endure those special indignities, such as humiliating examinations by groups of medical students, reserved for the less privileged and less articulate.

The rich also look upon medical care and health as commodities but they have enough money (that ultimate fetish) to buy as much of it as they want. Many pay extravagantly for care they consider superior (and which is certainly more comfortable), although physicians who overcharge (relatively speaking) for their services are not necessarily better than the rest. Many hospitals have "executive checkup" programs, which means that a structured arrangement exists for shunting the rich in ahead of the rest in the long lineups for various examinations.

Personal health has a price and is a commodity to be bartered on the marketplace in exchange for other commodities. When British coal miners struck for higher wages in late 1973, they brought forward the morbid effects of the work environment upon their health, and their increased mortality rates, as arguments, not to correct the appalling working conditions, but to strengthen the case for higher pay.[24] This medical alienation of workers is really a part of the alienation of work activity. Exploited physically as well as economically, they are obliged to choose between their pulmonary function and their pocketbooks.

Physicians, too, regard the health of their patients as a commodity, to be valued in comparison with other commodities. Thus patients are often categorized either as "interesting teaching material" or as "crocks", the latter being vulnerable to discharge from hospital earlier than their rate of recovery warrants, in the heartless interest of "freeing beds".

H.B. Waitzkin and B. Waterman, in their study *The Exploitation of Illness in Capitalist Society*, have included a discussion of patient alienation in their attempt to apply Marxian analysis to some of the problems in medicine. They maintain that, "By analogy with Marx's analysis, patients might be considered a unique social class."[25] While adding the qualification that the analogy with Marx's usage is not strictly comparable, they suggest that patients become "alienated through a . . . loss of control over [their bodies]".[26]

What should be clear from the foregoing analysis is that patients do not *become* alienated through loss of control over their bodies. They *are* alienated because they live in a society in which productive activity and interpersonal relations are alienated. That they lack control over their bodies in the medical context is an expression of their alienated relationship to health workers.*

Alienation of the medical student

Medical students are not a special class and do not experience a special alienation. As people who function in an alienated society, they experience as much alienation as many others. In particular, their alienation is manifested through the work experience and through the needs it gives rise to; thus their alienation is comparable to that of the physicians they emulate and eventually become. The alienation of medical students (and young physicians-in-training) does, however, have some noteworthy characteristics.

In the first place, alienated social relations are often a major reason for entering medical school: economic insecurity, competitiveness, family pressure to "succeed"; in short, all those expressions of a society that, in its basic economic relations, sets each person against every other. The idealism and human concern for others that so many medical students give as their reason for wanting to undertake the study of medicine are often stalking horses for these alienated needs and values. Such idealism is sufficiently superficial that little of it endures amidst the continuing bombardment of alienated experience that the student encounters in the medical school, in the hospital and in medical practice.

Alienation manifests itself in a number of ways in medical school: in the relationships between medical students (excessive competitiveness, sadomasochistic interaction); in their relationship to their "productive activity" (learning by rote to prepare for examinations rather than for medical practice, developing strategies in the early years to acquire appropriate letters of recommendation for subsequent training, burying themselves in their studies to the exclusion of all other activity, readily grasping the role and title of "Doctor" with which to mediate their other social interactions); and in relationship to the product of their activity (lack of sensitivity to the needs of their patients, failure to acquire the ability to communicate effectively with the poor, a tendency to specialize and to seek material wealth, even when this occurs at the expense of patients).

Medicine and the authoritarian personality

Authoritarianism: some background

The authoritarian personality is a character type that has been described in the course of psychoanalytic investigations by Wilhelm

Reich, Karen Horney and Erich Fromm, and has been the subject of important works by Max Horkheimer and Theodor Adorno, among others. It is a syndrome that combines in one person the seemingly contradictory strivings for both sadistic and masochistic interactions with others.

The sadomasochistic, or authoritarian, personality type should not be confused with the sadomasochistic "perversion", which relates to the abuse of the human body in the course of sexual activity. Sexual sadomasochism is thought to be an extreme manifestation of the far more prevalent character type.[27]

Authoritarian personalities long for relationships with others that are based on the dominance of one party over another, rather than for relationships in which participation is more equitable.[28] They relate to those around them in terms of the strengths or weaknesses of others relative to themselves. They are attracted to the extremes: those who are weak whom they can dominate, and those who are strong to whom they can submit.

Authoritarianism is a common but not inevitable feature of human relationships.[29] Why and when does it occur? Is it, perhaps, an inborn trait? Is it a function of some stimulus in the environments of certain people? Or is it a manifestation of problems within society as a whole?

The roots of present-day authoritarianism lie in two important developments of the Renaissance period: the rise of the capitalist mode of production and the emergence of the Protestant religions.* The new capitalist order freed a large number of people for the first time, setting them loose from the feudal bonds of subservience. Although capitalist society still distributed wealth inequitably, individuals became free agents to the extent they had the right to compete in the open marketplace for economic and social roles and positions. For many, however, the new order was an intimidating rather than liberating force. Insecurity generated by the sudden dislocations in people's lives helped shape a new human character, the psychological foundations upon which authoritarian institutions and relationships would be erected.[30]

Into the gap created between old and new ways of life also came the Protestant churches. They preached not only the affirmation of the individual and the right to relate directly to God without the necessary intervention of the Church or the Communion of the Saints, but also, and perhaps more importantly, a submission before God, the doctrine of subordination apparent in the writings of Martin Luther and John Calvin.*

People who felt insecure in the face of the tumultuous changes in society — this was particularly true of members of the middle class — welcomed the opportunity to submit before the authority of a religious doctrine that made life seem somewhat less complicated.* The religion rationalized the severing of their feudal bonds and "freed" them from some of the anxieties that accompanied the end of feudal servitude.

The embrace of Protestant doctrine by the members of the middle class had two important consequences for the socio-economic order. First, it promoted acquiescence in that order by people who were not really satisfied with it.* Second, it fostered the Protestant work ethic — the willingness and compulsion of some individuals to engage in unceasing hard work. This new preparedness to be productive in the marketplace predictably contributed to the acceleration of economic development.[31] In the end, Protestant ideology provided an escape for people in capitalist society. It allowed beleaguered citizens to cope with otherwise intolerable anxieties. They submitted themselves to the authority of God and, by engaging in unceasing effort, submerged in a "greater whole". These adjustments provided a kind of relief, particularly to the embattled middle class, but at the price of any independent and critical participation in their society.

Why is it that in modern society some people still long for authoritarian relationships? We have come a long way since the early days of capitalism, after all, and the power of the Protestant church has long since passed its peak. Yet there has been no concomitant decline in the prevalence of the authoritarian personality, although its expression has become more varied.

Authority in human relationships can be characterized as falling along a continuum between rational and irrational. Rational authority exists only for the mutual benefit of the parties involved, and tends to dissolve itself with the passage of time; good examples of this are sometimes found in student-teacher relationships. Irrational authority, on the other hand, is based on the exploitation of one person by another; relationships of this kind do not tend to dissolve, since their function is to satisfy an enduring and unhealthy psychological need.

Authority in the feudal era was almost totally irrational, since it promoted exploitation and prevented individual human development. While this sort of overt, oppressive authority is less evident in our era, other forms of authority have arisen in its place. Some of the new authorities are anonymous, meaning that they do not exist in law or in the power explicitly exerted by one over another. These anonymous authorities are to be found inside individuals, in the form of "common sense", faith, allegiance to a nation-state or to another institution — like medicine — or an internal compulsion to work. They can be just as irrational and oppressive as any feudal lord. Since they are not overt, however, their impact is not uniform throughout society: some individuals will be totally submissive before them, others hardly at all.

It has become extremely difficult for people to relate healthfully and spontaneously to their work, to their environment and to others. Society has developed dimensions and characteristics people cannot cope with and relate to humanely. We have lost both our sense of proportion and our identity. Not infrequently, we feel the need to conform to the expectations of others, to win their acceptance and thereby a modicum of security, whatever the cost in spontaneity and individuality.[32]

Thus some people who have been frustrated in the effort to relate in a positive, fulfilling way to the world accept a solution that not only falls short of satisfying their needs and fulfilling their aspirations, but is frequently incompatible with these ends. The solution, masochistic submission, seeks meaning for life in its very negation, in the "annihilation of the self".[33]

Is some degree of authoritarianism an inevitable consequence of what we call progress and the increasing complexity of our culture? According to Erich Fromm, who has devoted much of his career as a psychoanalyst to the examination of various manifestations of authoritarianism, societies based upon competitiveness and the exploitation of some individuals by others — including all major civilizations up until now — are largely to blame for the development of sadomasochistic traits in many of their citizens.*

In fact, we may assume that some degree of authoritarianism is present in most people. There are some individuals, however, in whom sadomasochistic or authoritarian traits predominate. Fromm found that about ten per cent of the population of Germany, just prior to the rise of Hitler, fell into this category, and that these people mostly belonged to the lower middle class. Like their counterparts in the early days of capitalism, members of this class were most anxious and least hopeful about the changes taking place in their society.

In an extensive study of authoritarian behaviour in the United States, T.W. Adorno and others proposed a somewhat different relationship between social class and authoritarianism: that the authoritarian personality is most likely to find expression "amongst those whose status differs markedly from that to which they aspire".[34] This is an attractive concept that one might be tempted to apply, for example, to the field of medicine. It is important to remember, however, that a class or group or individual whose expectations are frustrated will not always seek refuge in authoritarian interaction. For example, some people search out those situations within society that are less stifling and that allow for more humane and creative individual development.

The important difference between people who seek to escape their oppression and those who strive to overcome it lies in their attitude towards the possibility of change. Those who have lost hope that an oppressive situation can be altered, who fail to see conflicts and contradictions within society as the possible precursors of change, and who are so disturbed by the problems they face that the prospect of change is even more terrifying than their present state, will not seek liberating, anti-authoritarian solutions to their problems. In a futile bid to avoid an unbearable fate with no apparent alternatives, they may submit to irrational authorities and seek to hold power over others. Thus are they driven even further from any conception of improving their plight, either as individuals or as members of a group or class.

Other factors operating at the individual level may either forestall or generate authoritarian behaviour. The person whose social situation is not fulfilling may be protected from a sense of "vital powerlessness" by a meaningful family life; similarly a person whose home situation is not fulfilling may find relief elsewhere. It is the unfortunate people (and in some circumstances, classes) with no alternative source of nourishment for their psycho-social needs who are likely to seek an outlet for their frustrations and an escape from their fears in authoritarianism.[35]

Conversely, persons who have strong tendencies towards authoritarianism are unlikely to express them if discouraged from so doing by their social environment.[36] However, such persons may well seek out, consciously or otherwise, those situations within society in which authoritarianism can be most easily and completely expressed.

Authoritarianism in medicine

As we've seen earlier in this book, authoritarian behaviour can be observed at most stages of medical education and in almost all areas of hospital medical practice. The earliest manifestations appear in the prospective physician well before entry into medical school. Ever-increasing numbers of young people are looking to the institution and the profession of medicine as a way of escaping from the pressure and competitiveness almost all members of society face in their daily lives; they seek to escape this reality in a way that is at once socially acceptable and psychologically bearable. Many medical school applicants approach the prospect of a medical career uncritically and unrealistically, expecting that it will transform and give meaning to a less than satisfactory existence. All too willingly, they submit before the authority of the institution of medicine, submerging themselves in it, but inescapably forfeiting part of their own identities in doing so.*

Once in medical school they continue to submit. Motivated as many of them are by a desire to escape from the social, economic and psychological problems of their lives, they suffer from an irrational fear of failing, of falling back into the ranks of the anxiety-fraught masses. For many students, the response to this fear is to work and to study compulsively and continually, very much in the way early Protestants tried to escape from their anxieties through the hard work that would, presumably, predict their fate.

The "game of graded promotions" and others like it keep students busy enough to ignore "the forces which shape their cosmos". They begin to react to their environment by relating sadistically to classmates when the opportunity presents itself. In this, the most authoritarian students lead the way, setting the mood for the rest.

When medical students leave the classroom behind to begin the clinical phase of their training, a whole new world — the hospital — opens up to them. Insecure in the profound complexity and eerie oppressiveness of the place, they set out to define their role within it. They often feel ill at ease and unable to relate to the institution as a whole, an institution as overwhelming to them as it is to patients. The students' easiest course is to accept the role that has already been defined for them in considerable detail, beginning with the quite inappropriate title "Doctor".

Their relationships with patients give them lots of opportunities to develop any authoritarian tendencies they may have brought with them to the hospital. Their relationships with most others are defined by their identity as physicians and by their stage of training. They will acquire no more important "clinical skill" than the ability to see themselves, their institution and those around them through the eyes of the physician.

As in any authoritarian situation, it is possible to relate in two directions: towards those who are stronger and towards those who are weaker. For physicians-in-training, authority rests for the most part with physicians ranking higher in the hospital hierarchy. They submit readily before them, identifying totally with an institution defined in terms of superiors ("I am working on Smith's service", etc.). They accept without question the authority of their bosses, intellectual as well as juridical, not infrequently when their acquiescence is harmful to a patient. They also accept without too much resistance the authority of some others who are able to dominate them, such as head nurses. But everyone else is a potential target for the exercise of irrational authority.

The more convincingly they portray their professional role, sought in the first place because of an inability to master an uncertain and hostile world in any other way, the more power they are able to exercise over others (in personal life as well as the hospital). But the weaker they become in reality, because they drown in their institutional identity. Not only do physicians-in-training learn to tolerate relationships in the hospital that had once seemed so hostile and alien, but they also come at length to regard them as more natural and desirable than any other set of relationships.

Ultimately, their professional identity fails to provide them with what they wanted most of all. As they go along, they become *less* confident of their ability to relate as themselves to the world around them and to others in it. As they progress, they dare less and less to challenge the status quo in the hospital or the medical school in any significant way; their masochistic submission is thereby compounded. To whatever extent their initial decision to study medicine was motivated by "vital powerlessness", manifested as authoritarian behaviour, they become that much weaker as they proceed through studies and training, and even more dependent upon sadistic and masochistic interaction.

And, as we've seen, very often the authoritarianism of physicians is encouraged by parallel tendencies in others around them. Operating room nurses who submit before the authority of their surgeon-bosses on the one hand and subject neophyte medical students to humiliation and abuse on the other, are authoritarian too. Nurses who are not in a position to exercise authority over physicians may turn instead to abuse of orderlies and others who rank below them in the hierarchy, while acquiescing willingly before all medical authority.

Even patients can participate in the authority structure through what sociologists call the "sick role", or "sickness behaviour", seeking to escape unbearable pressures and anxieties in their daily lives by submitting before the institution of medicine and the authority of its practitioners.

There is no single cause of authoritarianism and it is probably not possible to quantify the presence of authoritarian behaviour in medicine, simply because appropriate techniques of measurement do not exist. It is safe to say that it is of sufficient importance to merit systematic analysis. What must be explained in any event is why authoritarian personalities and destructive, authoritarian behaviour should be a significant reality in this presumably humane, "liberal" profession.

It should be pointed out first that some of the authority is quite rational and appropriate, as in the case of a very ill person who is incapable of making a decision about therapy, particularly in an emergency situation. But if the allocation of authority in the physician-patient encounter were entirely rational, the power relation would dissolve as the patient's health improved and he or she became better able to participate in decisions about care. Because it is irrational, however, the physician's authority does not evaporate. It stems not from any therapeutic necessity, but from the desire of the physician to hold power over others, and from the willingness of the patient to submit.

Why should some people strive to subject themselves, through a sick role, to the authority of others? For one thing, the submission before religious doctrine and the authority of God are no longer tenable expressions of masochistic longings. So the ready availability of a more credible institution that seeks submission — the institution of medicine — is an acceptable alternative. For some persons, medicine has proved an effective opiate, both literally and figuratively.

The authoritarianism of physicians is influenced by a number of factors. Some people are no doubt drawn to a medical career at least in part because of the great scope it offers to those who like to make authority the focus of relationships. But if, among medical school applicants, there exists a disproportionate concentration of authoritarians, it is no less true that the selection process at most schools tends to favour just these individuals. Those who have submerged themselves completely in their studies, to the exclusion of all other concerns, are more likely to be assessed as demonstrating the stability and certainty about a career (and are much more likely to have high marks) so attractive to admissions committees.

Once it has them in its clutches, the medical school immediately sets about fostering insecurity and uncertainty in its students. It encourages them to develop their authoritarian proclivities, sometimes specifically rewarding them for doing so, or punishing them for failing to act "professionally". The same process occurs among nursing students.

Even persons with minimal authoritarian tendencies can be affected. Subjected to the irrational authority of others, student nurses or physicians may feel so threatened that they are driven into authoritarian patterns through self-defence.*

All these trends continue into clinical training. The situations in which physicians-to-be first encounter patients in a therapeutic role are often those in which the patients are sickest and weakest, and hence least able to participate. Such extreme situations are not typical of medical interaction, but the power they enjoy in these initial encounters may whet their appetite for more control over others. As one group of researchers found, students develop an image of the Ideal Physician, characterized by extroversion, slight emotion, thorough dominance and handsome appearance, while coming to view the patient in the opposite terms: introverted, emotional, weak-willed and ugly.[37]

That many people behave in authoritarian ways in such structured and oppressive circumstances is not surprising. Their numbers would be far fewer were it not that our society not only permits, but also approves of and actively encourages authoritarian relationships.* Even so, there are many degrees of authoritarianism, and many people who are negligibly authoritarian if at all. As Erich Fromm says:

[N]ot every situation where a person or a group has uncontrolled power over another generates sadism. Many — perhaps most — parents, prison guards, school teachers, and bureaucrats are not sadistic. For any number of reasons, the character structure of many individuals is not conducive to the development of sadism even under circumstances that offer an opportunity for it. Persons who have a dominantly life-furthering character will not easily be seduced by power. But it would be a dangerous oversimplification if I were to classify people into only two groups: the sadistic devils and the non-sadistic saints. What matters is the intensity of the sadistic passion within the character structure of a given person.[38]

In medicine, degrees of authoritarianism can be reflected in the choice of a specialty: the most authoritarian will enter training programs which offer the most opportunities for sadistic and masochistic interaction. Needless to say, there are many exceptions to any prevailing pattern but, in general, as we've seen earlier, surgery offers greater attractions to the authoritarian than most specialties while the opposite is true of pediatrics.

The most hopeful evidence that human relationships can be freed of authoritarian destructiveness is the fact that some people, in medicine as elsewhere, contrive not to be "seduced by power". But it should also be clear that to truly accomplish this freeing of human relationships, more than our medical schools and hospitals will have to be changed.

Alienation and authoritarianism are serious problems — in medicine as elsewhere. When we recognize that these problems are rooted in an oppressive social order we are not likely to be deluded into believing that they can be corrected with cosmetics. Notwithstanding the attempts of Ivan Illich and some others to indict medicine for society's ills, and the efforts of others to identify the One Problem that stands in the way of more humane medical care, significant change in medicine can only come as part of a more general transformation of society itself.

Notes

page 182: For example, the number of hospital employees in the United States increased from 662,000 in 1950 to 1,824,000 in 1969. (J. and B. Ehrenreich, "Hospital Workers: a case study of the new working class", *Monthly Review*, Jan. 1975, pp12-27.)

page 183a: Another important consideration is that alienation is not limited to the factory floor and those other settings for productive activity that usually come to mind as places in which people can invest their labour. While he never published an exhaustive list, Marx did say on one occasion that "religion, family, state, law, morality, science, art, etc." are all "particular modes [or forms] of production" in which capitalist relations can be expressed. (K. Marx, *The Economic and Philosophic Manuscripts of 1844*, trans. M. Mulligan [New York: International Publishers, 1964] p136.) Some people objectify at least some of their labour in each of these institutions. More importantly, these are man-made institutions in society, and it is through them that much social interaction takes place. None of this is meant to deny the essential nature of capitalist production, in the economic sense, as a fundamental expression of alienation to which all others are vitally linked.

183b: All people are, to at least some degree, alienated in capitalist society — and not only because they work for capitalists. "The whole of human servitude is involved in the relation of the worker to production, and every relation of servitude is but a modification and consequence of this relation." (Marx, *The Economic and Philosophic Manuscripts of 1844*, p116.)

page 184a: On the one hand, were people not thus alienated in their relationships to others, the alienation of labour could not occur. On the other hand:

[I]*f the products of his labour, his labour objectified, is for him an alien, hostile, powerful object independent of him, then his position towards it is such that someone else is master of this object, someone who is alien, hostile, powerful and independent of him ...*

Through estranged labour man not only creates his relationship to the object and the act of production as to men that are alien and hostile to him; he also creates the relationship in which other men stand to his production and to his product, and the relationship in which he stands to these other men. (K. Marx, *The Economic and Philosophic Manuscripts of 1844*, p116.)

184b: *For the time being, there remains . . . the "reversed" form in which the social relations of man are now reflected as mere relations of things. There remain unchanged . . . and there will remain as long as the products of labour are produced as commodities, all the fetish-categories of bourgeois economics: commodity, money, capital, wage-labour, increasing and decreasing total value of production and of export, profit-making capacity of industries, credits, etc.; in short, all that which Marx in his philosophic phase called "human self-alienation", and in his scientific phase, "fetishism of commodity production".* (K. Korsch, *Karl Marx* [New York, Wiley and Sons, 1938], p150.)

page 185: When discussing the problems of such workers with a colleague on one occasion, I was given the following account of the work situation of a particular orderly: "This man has a lot of pride and dignity," my fellow intern explained, "but he never fails to say 'Yes, doctor', when responding to interns or residents who are half his age. He tolerates occasional verbal abuse, but handles himself very well, working hard and doing a good job. He certainly earns his pay, and he disposes of it scrupulously. When he finishes work, he changes into a spotless suit; his shoes are always polished, his clothes never wrinkled. He and his wife run a dancing school in the evenings, and they supplement his income in that way. Over a number of years, they have accumulated a considerable amount of money. They live quite comfortably, and someday he will be able to quit his job and live off his savings. How can you say this man is oppressed?"

However oppressed the orderly felt himself to be, my friend described rather succinctly the alienation of productive activity which that man was experiencing, in a way that applies to many other health workers.

page 186a: Even when the assembly line is made less rigid, as in the recent experiments in some automobile plants, it is only done to defuse the discontent experienced by workers, who have not lost all their inner drive to express their human potentiality. It is ironic that industrial psychologists have been able to show that efficiency in a factory can be improved by an intervention in the form of an experiment, not because the intervention necessarily improves working conditions but because someone is demonstrating to the workers that they consider them and their work important enough to focus some attention upon them — the so-called "Hawthorne Effect". (See J.A.C. Brown, *The Social Psychology of Industry* [Harmondsworth, Middlesex: Pelican Books Inc., 1954], pp69-96.)

186b: Nursing is a career frequently undertaken by women of the lower middle class and the working class in order to gain upward social mobility. In this sense, it is not a spontaneous realization of self, but a class-mediated expression of a need external to the individual.

The sale of labour power to a medical institution is considered to be sacrosanct, and more significant than most sales of commodities. Society looks upon attempts by nurses and other health workers to withdraw their services as particularly reprehensible. Thus does the medical institution claim "a title and a right to the labour and the surplus-labour of others", a sophistication that is, according to Marx, characteristic of capitalist production.

(Other 'public service' workers share this unhappy distinction with nurses.)

page 187a: Asked why he had turned down a $30,000 a year appointment at a university hospital in favour of private practice, a physician I know replied: "Medicine is a business. For myself it is a very good business. You cannot support a nice home and a family and send your four kids to private schools on $30,000 a year."

187b: This is particularly true in the hospital, where the contributions to "care" of many physicians are virtually anonymous and each is, in a sense, expendable, in spite of having had considerable training. This is certainly a far cry from the situation in which a person makes a personal mark on the world. Nonetheless, the hospital claims night labour and extremely long hours from many physicians in the fulfilment of their responsibilities. Thus, in the hospital setting at least, physicians function largely as adjuncts to machines, totally responsive to and dependent upon them; the hospital, on the other hand, can make considerable, and sometimes unreasonable, demands on the people who are physicians in order to fulfil its "human" needs. A narrative illustration of this point is provided by Robin Cook in his book *Year of the Intern. (op. cit.)*

page 188a: Far from being able to contemplate themselves in a world that is the expression of their productive activity, physicians use material commodities (wealth, social status, power over others) to buffer themselves from a world over which they have little control, and which is so "out of joint".

188b: Other factors that contribute to their contentedness are the social dividends that work and position provide, and the work experience itself, which is more meaningful and less alienated than that of many other workers (at least in the abstract, having some significance beyond the provision of a pay packet). That physicians are usually more comfortable in their alienation than the majority of workers is evidenced by the nearly universal tendency of physicians to mediate most, if not all, their social interaction through their identities as physicians. Physicians regularly accept the definition of themselves and their possibilities embodied in the title "Doctor", and do not often seek to exceed the confines of this role, either inside or outside of their usual productive activity.

page 189a: Of course, if a product is a result of alienated productive activity, it too will be alienated. But Marx saw special significance in the product itself and deemed it worthy of separate analysis as a focus of alienation.

189b: There are other ways in which workers are subjugated to the product they do not control. The specifications to which a product is produced, and the ways in which it is promoted (often designed to create an artificial need for it) determine the uses to which it will be put and, hence, the way of life of the worker. For example, when motor vehicles are designed to hold four to six passengers, most people travel to work in private vehicles. Hence the attitude of all too many people in Los Angeles to the lack of adequate public transit facilities: "Who needs it? The freeways are so good!" Similarly, the promotion of snowmobiles in the mass media displaces the importance of their use to those who must travel where there are no roads, and transforms them into luxury items to be desired by all (to the advantage of the capitalist, of course).

Thus are people alienated from their products, and not only because products are produced by alienated labour. The product turns the tables on the worker (who would make a personal mark on the world through it) and "his life no longer belongs to himself but to the object". (See K. Marx, *A Contribution to the Critique of Political Economy*, trans. M. Mulligan [New York: International Publishers, 1970], p108.)

189c: When a health service is provided to them — even *their* health service — someone else usually profits, directly or indirectly.

page 190a: An example of this is the kidney specialist who advocates an extensive battery of tests on each patient with hypertension, even though the knowledge provided by the results of these tests does not make it possible to provide better treatment. The physician's interest is to focus attention on the occasional association of hypertension with kidney dysfunction, which is quite independent of the patient's objective interest: to have blood pressure controlled.

190b: In other words, cigarette advertising and the dirty air spewing forth from the factories and automobiles are not going to disappear through the professional endeavours of the lung specialist.

190c: Nor do patients have very much more control over the condition of their lungs than does the physician.

190d: Thus do we have the almost comical spectacle, in the treatment of hypertension, of the physician who keeps increasing the dosage of the prescribed medicine but fails to lower the blood pressure of the patient because the latter is not taking any of the medication.

190e: A slightly different conflict of interest between worker and product is represented by the decision that interns or residents must make about how much time to spend with a patient. Interns are on salary, and a rather paltry one at that (or at least it was, until recently). They have very long working hours and put in many nights on duty, an experience that taxes them physically as well as emotionally. Yet, they have a certain amount of latitude in determining how much work they do. What time to leave the hospital on nights off? How much time to spend answering a call and dealing with a problem that arises in the middle of the night when they could otherwise be obtaining some much-needed sleep? Since the staffing of the hospital is rarely sufficient to assure adequate care unless the interns and residents over-extend themselves, house officers are faced with a choice between their own relative health, well-being and well-rounded development, and the health and well-being of the patient, the product of their activity, which is frequently an "alien force" inconsistent with their own interests.

page 191a: Thus are rotations in community hospitals considered excellent experiences for the junior house staff, because these physicians-in-training are given the opportunity to exercise greater responsibility there, notwithstanding the quality of care, which is probably inferior.

191b: That a person's product becomes an object is true in any advanced society, alienated or not, in which there is a productive process. That it can exist independently of the worker is a particular characteristic of an alienated society, in which the product is built according to the specifications of another person or group of persons and, once produced, is not the worker's to use. (See B. Ollman, *Alienation,* [Cambridge: Cambridge University Press, 1971], pp144-146, and I. Meszaros, *Marx's Theory of Alienation,* [London: The Merlin Press, 1970], pp173-174.)

page 193: This brings up an important consideration of the relationship between medical practice and alienation. If the life activity (work) of the person who is a patient is but a means to life, that life is alienated, and even the most humanely delivered medical care can only accomplish the prolongation and amelioration of an alienated existence. That is not to say that alienated people are not worthy of medical care: of course they are, but health workers would be able to make a much richer and more valuable contribution to their patients' well being if the lives they were helping involved more than just the pursuit of the means to life.

In such a situation, health workers would be able to do that which is most fulfilling: to create the conditions necessary for existence, as far as possible free of disease and pain, so that they and others might best be able to contemplate themselves in a world people had built.

page 194a: Another aspect of patient alienation in relation to medicine is a direct correlate of work experience. A person who is fed up with work may come to a medical facility feigning illness, hoping to deceive the physician and thereby obtain a medical excuse to avoid going to work. There is another way in which encounters in medicine can reflect the prevailing mode of production and of socio-economic interaction: a person who is exploited and denied dignity in daily life and work may approach the physician for the companionship and the attention which is not forthcoming in others parts of life; in so doing, this person may make undue demands on the available time of health workers, whose responsibilities and priorities lie elsewhere. (Every hospital's Emergency Room has a collection of "society's rejects" who troop through regularly in search of fulfilment of their alienated needs for companionship.)

The inconsistency with which patients follow the physician's recommendations and take the prescribed medications is yet another manifestation of patient alienation which plagues medical practice. Many of the reasons why people fail to comply are predictable outcomes of their alienated social relations (poverty, economic and social crises in the household, the inability of the physician to spend the time necessary to educate the patient properly about his disease and the treatment, etc.) (See J.R. Caldwell, "The dropout problem in antihypertensive treatment", *Journal of Chronic Diseases* 22, 1970, pp579-82.)

194b: Thus are the social and human roots of commodities obscured. Objects are seen as "natural" and immune to change in social relations:

[We regard a commodity as having] *a "natural" price, a relation to money and other commodities independent of the human factors involved . . . [which] is taken as a non-social quality of the commodity on a par with its physical character, shoes have openings for feet and cost five dollars a pair.* (B. Ollman, *Alienation*, p199).

Thus it is also frequently said that money can "earn" a profit for its owner through investments when, in reality, profit is derived from the activity of other people. Similarly, a worker may look upon technology as the oppressor, when the true source of oppression is in the organization of society and hence the factory.

Bourgeois society thus deludes itself about the place of the commodity in human relations. According to Marx:

[The commodity has become] *a mysterious thing, simply because in it the social character of men's labour appears to them as an objective character stamped upon the product of that labour because the relation of the producers to the sum total of their labour is presented to them as a social relation, not existing between themselves, but between the products of their labour.* (K. Marx, *Capital*, Vol. 1, New York, International Publishers, 1967, p72.)

194c: It may seem obvious, in the abstract, that fad diets and vitamin supplements, for example, being of no proven efficacy, are in no way part of the natural order of things; yet when health has become a commodity, it is increasingly the norm for people to suppose that good health can be bought in these forms off the supermarket shelf, to be then accepted as natural constituents of everyday life.

page 195: To advocate "free" medical care, as many proponents of the welfare state tend to do, is to fall into the trap of treating medical care as a commodity which has a particular price, rather than as a right of all members of the society.

page 196: Likewise, the concept of patients as a special class is inconsistent with Marxian analysis and quite unnecessary for an understanding of their alienation and exploitation.

page 197a: Much of the discussion in this section is derived from the work of Erich Fromm, and especially from his book *Escape From Freedom* (New York: Holt, Rinehart and Winston, 1941).

197b: Martin Luther taught that, while there is no natural social order there is, so to speak, a natural spiritual one, and while no man is by right the master of another, neither can any man consider himself his own master. Calvin preached that man's fate is completely beyond his control, is predetermined and is inalterable. He contended that some are predestined by God for grace and others for eternal damnation:

We are not our own; therefore, neither our reason nor our will should predominate in our deliberations and actions. We are not our own; therefore, let us, as far as possible, forget ourselves and all things that are ours. On the contrary, we are

God's; to him, let us live and die. (J. Calvin, *Institutes of the Christian Religion,* trans. J. Allen, [Philadelphia, 1928] Book III, Chap. 7, p1; see also Fromm, *Escape From Freedom,* pp40-102.)

page 198a: This doctrine did give the members of the middle class a sense of security. In a society in which important aspects of their existence were beyond their control, people could be assured that at least one thing was certain: their eternal fate in the determination of which they were completely at the mercy of God. Those who were destined to go to heaven would, of course, prove worthy through hard work. Thus did men, in an attempt to predict their predetermined fate, adopt the Protestant ethic of hard work.

page 198b: According to Fromm:

They taught [the member of the middle class] *that by fully accepting his power-lessness and the evil of his nature, by considering his whole life an atonement for his sins, by his utmost self-humiliation, and also by unceasing effort, he could overcome his doubt and his anxiety; that by complete submission he could be loved by God and could at least hope to belong to those whom God had decided to save. Protestantism was the answer to the human needs of the frightened, uprooted, and isolated individual who had to orient and to relate himself to a new world.* (Fromm, *Escape From Freedom,* p101.)

page 199: [T]*he power through which one group exploits and keeps down another tends to generate sadism in the controlling group, even though there will be many individual exceptions.*

A society based on exploitative control also exhibits other predictable features. It tends to weaken the independence, critical thinking, and productivity of those submitted to it . . .

. . . Sadism is one of the answers to the problem of being born human when better ones are not attainable. The experience of absolute control over another human being, of omnipotence as far as he, she, or it is concerned, creates the illusion of transcending the limitations of human existence, particularly for one whose real life is deprived of productivity and joy . . . It is the transformation of the impotence into the experience of omnipotence. (E. Fromm, *The Anatomy of Human Destructive-ness* [New York: Holt, Rinehart and Winston, 1973], pp290-291.)

page 201: They do this prior to their entry into medical school by identifying themselves as "pre-med" students.

page 204a: See Erich Fromm's discussion of defensive aggression in *The Anatomy of Human Destructiveness.*

204b: Medicine is an (almost) unique institution that offers a channel for authoritarian tendencies to patients, physicians and other health workers alike. While it is difficult to conceive of a society in which medicine did not exist as some sort of institution, it is by no means inevitable that it would always be a forum for authoritarianism, although that would probably be the case in any society based on the exercise by some of irrational authority over others.

References

Preface

1. I.D. Illich, *Medical Nemesis: The expropriation of health* (New York: Pantheon, 1975).

2. M.F.W. Goss, R.M. Battistella, J. Colombotos, E. Friedson, D.C. Riedel, "Social organization and control in medical work: a call for research", *Medical Care* 15, no.5, supplement 1-10 (May 1977).

3. B. Brecht, "Writing the truth: five difficulties", reprinted in B. Brecht, *Galileo*, ed. E. Bentley, trans. C. Laughton (New York: Grove Press, 1966), p141.

Chapter One: Getting In

1. S. Judek, *Medical Manpower in Canada: Royal Commission on Health Services* (Ottawa: Queen's Printer, 1964).

2. H.H. Gee, "The student's view of the medical school admissions process", in H.H. Gee, J.T. Cowles, "The Appraisal of Applicants to Medical School", *Journal of Medical Education* 32, no.10, part 2 (1957): 110-152; and H.C. Gough, W.B. Hall, "A comparison of medical students from medical and nonmedical families", *Journal of Medical Education* 52 (1977): 541-547.

3. B.R. Blishen, *Doctors and Doctrines* (Toronto: University of Toronto Press, 1969), p33.

4. S.G. Wolf, "I can't afford a B", *New England Journal of Medicine* 299 (1978): 949-950.

5. *Los Angeles Times*, 14 July, 1976, pII-1.

6. "Medical Education in the United States", *Journal of the American Medical Association* 238 (1977): 2771-2772.

7. *Los Angeles Times*, 9 November, 1976, (editorial) pII-4.

8. "Medical Education in the United States, 1972-3", *Journal of the Ameri-*

can Medical Association 226 (1973): 913-914.

9. *New York Times,* 14 November, 1976, p26.

10. V. Navarro, "Women in health care", *New England Journal of Medicine* 292 (1975): 398-402.

11. M.C. Howell, "What medical schools teach about women", *New England Journal of Medicine* 291 (1974): 304-307.

12. J. Abourbih, "The admission of women to the McGill medical school", *McGill Medical Journal* 40, no. 2, 3 (1971): 22-24.

13. F.J. Ingelfinger, "Doctor women", *New England Journal of Medicine* 291 (1974): 303-304.

14. A Chesney, *The Johns Hopkins School of Medicine: A Chronicle,* vol. 1, chap. 8 (Baltimore: Johns Hopkins Press, 1943).

15. The account that follows is from J. Abourbih, *op.cit.*

16. W. Osler, "Presidential address to the Canadian Medical Association, Chatham, Ont., 1885", *Canadian Medical and Surgical Journal* 14 (1885): 129-155.

17. C. Nadelson, M.T. Notman, "The woman physician", *Journal of Medical Education* 47 (1972): 176-183.

18. M.C. Howell, *op.cit.*

19. E. Ramey, "An interview with Dr. Estelle Ramey", *Perspectives in Biology and Medicine* 14 (1971): 424-431.

20. H.M. Spiro, "Visceral viewpoints: Myths and Mirths — Women in Medicine", *New England Journal of Medicine* 292 (1975): 354-356.

21. A. Flexner, *Medical Education in the United States and Canada* (Boston: D.B. Updike, The Merrymount Press, 1910).

22. R. Stevens, *American Medicine and the Public Interest* (New Haven: Yale University Press, 1971), pp66-70.

23. *Ibid.,* p67.

24. *Ibid.,* p15.

25. *Ibid.,* p25.

26. *Ibid.,* pp69-70.

27. H.S. Pritchett, "Introduction" to A. Flexner, *op.cit.,* pxi.

28. R. Stevens, *op.cit.,* pp364-365.

29. H.S. Pritchett, *op.cit.,* pxiv (emphasis added).

30. A. Flexner, *op.cit.,* pp15-17.

31. *Ibid.,* p17.

32. *Ibid.,* p15.

33. *Ibid.,* p150.

34. *Ibid.,* p21.

35. R. Stevens, *op.cit.,* pp71-73.

Chapter Two: Call Me Doctor

1. D. Rubinstein, "Stimulation of positive attitudes on biochemistry by incorporation of clinical presentations", *Journal of Medical Education* 47 (1972): 198-202.

2. G.R. Bernard, "Prosection demonstrations as substitutes for conventional human gross anatomy laboratory", *Journal of Medical Education* 47 (1972): 724-728.

3. R.C.A. Hunter, R.H. Prince, A.E. Schwartzman, "Comments on emotional disturbances in a medical undergraduate population", *Canadian Medical Association Journal* 83 (1961): 989-992.

4. F.L. McGuire, "Psycho-social studies of medical students: a critical review", *Journal of Medical Education* 41 (1966): 424-445.

5. E. Fromm, *Escape From Freedom* (New York: Holt, Rinehart and Winston, 1941), pp92-93.

6. "Medical Education in the United States, 1976-7", *Journal of American Medical Association* 238 (1977): 2774-2776.

7. D. Coburn, "Perceived sources of stress among first year medical students", *Journal of Medical Education* 50 (1975): 589-595.

8. Doctor X, *Intern* (New York: Harper and Row, 1965; Fawcett Crest edition, Greenwich, Conn.).

9. W. Nolen, *The Making of a Surgeon* (New York: Random House, 1970).

10. D. Bell, *A Time to be Born* (New York: William Morrow and Co., 1974).

11. R. Cook, *Year of the Intern* (New York: Harcourt, Brace, Jovanovitch, 1972; Signet edition, 1973).

12. *Ibid.*, p70.

13. Doctor X, *op.cit.*, p279.

14. R. Cook, *op.cit.*, pp178-179.

15. *Ibid.*, p125.

16. *Ibid.*, pp47,189.

17. G.R. Bernard, *op.cit.*, pp724-728.

18. H.S. Becker, B. Geer, E.C. Hughes, A.L. Strauss, *Boys in White* (Chicago: University of Chicago Press, 1961), pp92-184.

19. J.R. Wingard, J.W. Williamson, "Grades as predictors of physicians' career performance: an evaluative literature review", *Journal of Medical Education* 48 (1973): 311-320.

20. I.D. Illich, *Deschooling Society* (New York: Harper and Row; Harrow Books, 1971), p63.

21. *Ibid.*, pp54-56.

22. *Ibid.*, p74.

23. Health/PAC, "The student health organization: bringing it all back home", in B. Ehrenreich, J. Ehrenreich (eds.), *The American Health Em-*

pire: Power, Profits and Politics (New York: Random House, 1970), pp242-252.

24. R.J. Bazell, "Health radicals: crusade to shift medical power to the people", *Science* 173 (August 6, 1971), pp506-509.

25. J. Finley, "Creating a flexible medical curriculum", *McGill Medical Journal* 40, no.2,3 (1971): pp29-30.

26. R. Seidenberg, "Drug advertising and perception of mental illness", *Mental Hygiene* 55, no. 1 (Jan. 1971): pp21-31.

27. M. Mintz, "The stuff doctors read", *The Progressive* (April 1969), pp28-32; and M. Silverman, "The epidemiology of drug promotion", *International Journal of Health Services* 7, no.2 (1977): 157-165.

28. N.V. Peale, *The Power of Positive Thinking* (Englewood Cliffs, N.J.: Prentice-Hall, Inc., 1952; Fawcett Crest edition, 1962), p24.

29. G. Psathas, "The fate of idealism in nursing school", *Journal of Health and Social Behaviour* 9 (1968): 58-64.

30. R.D. Laing, "The mystification of experience", in R.D. Laing, *The Politics of Experience and The Bird of Paradise* (New York: Pantheon, 1967), p61.

31. E. Fromm, *op.cit.,* p162.

Chapter Three: On Receiving Knowledge

1. H.S. Becker, B. Geer, E.C. Hughes, A.L. Strauss, *Boys in White* (Chicago: University of Chicago Press, 1961), pp92-184.

2. *Ibid.,* p173.

3. *Ibid.,* pp120-121, 174-175.

4. K. Marx, *The Economic and Philosophic Manuscripts of 1844,* trans. M. Mulligan (New York: International Publishers, 1964), pp108, 110-111.

5. S.B. Langfeld, "Hypertension, deficient care of the medically served", *Annals of Internal Medicine* 78 (1973 pp19-23.

6. I.D. Illich, *Deschooling Society* (New York: Harper and Row; Harrow Books, 1971), p129.

7. K. Marx, *op.cit.,* p147.

Chapter Four: Doctors, Nurses and Students

1. V. Navarro, "The political economy of medical care; an explanation of the composition, nature and function of the present health sector of the United States", *International Journal of Health Services* 5, no.1 (1975): 65-94.

2. F. Gross, "The emperor's clothes syndrome", *New England Journal of Medicine* 285 (1971): 863.

3. W.A. Nolen, *The Making of a Surgeon* (New York: Random House, 1970), ppxiii-xiv.

4. *Ibid.*, p228.

5. *Ibid.*, pp91, 52-53.

6. *Ibid.*, p241.

7. See especially, Doctor X, *Intern* (New York: Harper and Row, 1965; Fawcett Crest edition); and W.A. Nolen, *op.cit.*

8. L.I. Stein, "The Doctor-nurse game", *Archives of General Psychiatry* 16 (1967): 699-703.

9. Gene, Lucy, Sue, Ellen and Eileen, "Woman hospital workers", *Science for the People* (Sept. 1974), pp12-14.

10. L.I. Stein, *op.cit.*

11. W.A. Nolen, *op.cit.*, p217.

12. *Ibid.*

13. L.I. Stein, *op.cit.*

14. *Ibid.*

15. See L. Richter, E. Richter, "Nurses in fiction", *American Journal of Nursing* 74, no.3 (1974): 1280-1281.

16. C.B. Gale, "Walking in the aides' shoes", *American Journal of Nursing* 73, no.4 (1973): 628-631.

17. V. Navarro, "Women in health care", *New England Journal of Medicine* 292 (1975): 398-402.

18. See also R. Milliband, *The State in Capitalist Society* (New York: Basic Books, 1969).

19. Gene, Lucy, Sue, Ellen and Eileen, *op.cit.*

20. V. Navarro, *op.cit.*

21. *Ibid.*

22. *Ibid.*

23. B. Ehrenreich, D. English, *Witches, Midwives and Nurses: A history of women healers* (Old Westbury, New York: The Feminist Press, 1975), pp6-18.

24. *Ibid.*, pp34-35.

25. *Ibid.*, p3.

26. V. Navarro, *op. cit.*

Chapter Five: Just What the Doctor Ordered

1. W. Nolen, *The Making of a Surgeon* (New York: Random House, 1970), p228.

2. Susan Sontag, "Fascinating Fascism", *New York Review of Books*, 22 no.1 (Feb. 6, 1975): 23-30.

3. M.S. Davis, "Variance in patients' compliance with doctors' orders: analysis of congruence between survey responses and results of empirical investigations", *Journal of Medical Education* 41 (1966): 1037-1048.

4. E. Friedson, *Profession of Medicine, a Study of the Sociology of Applied Knowledge* (New York: Dodd Mead and Co., 1973), p345.

5. *Ibid.*, pp307-308

6. A. Ordonez Plaja, L.M. Cohen, J. Samora, "La comunicacion entre el medico y el paciente en las consultas externas", *Educacion Medica y Salud* 3 (1969): 217-257.

7. K. Lennane, R.J. Lennane, "Alleged psychogenic disorders of women; a possible manifestation of sexual prejudice", *New England Journal of Medicine* 288: 288-292.

8. M.C. Howell, "What medical schools teach about women", *New England Journal of Medicine* 291 (1974): 304-307.

9. E. Frankfurt, *Vaginal Politics* (New York: Quadrangle, 1972), p19.

10. T. Parsons, *The Social System* (New York: The Free Press, 1951), pp428-479; and A. Segall, "The sick role concept: understanding illness behaviour", *Journal of Health and Social Behaviour* 17 (1976): 163-170.

11. H.B. Waitzkin, B. Waterman, *The Exploitation of Illness in Capitalist Society* (Indianapolis: Bobbs-Merrill, 1974), pp33-65.

12. M. Shapiro, "The patient should decide", *McGill Daily*, March 19, 1974, pp6-7; W.V. Slack, "The patient's right to decide", *The Lancet* 2 (1977): 240; S.H. Imbus, B.E. Zawacki, "Autonomy for burned patients when survival is unprecedented", *New England Journal of Medicine* 297 (1977): 308-311; E.J. Cassell, "Autonomy and ethics in action", *New England Journal of Medicine* 297 (1977): 333-334; and C.E. Lewis, M.A. Lewis, A. Lorimer, B.B. Palmer, "Child-initiated care: The utilization of school nursing services by chilfren in an 'adult-free' system", *Pediatrics* 60 (1977): 499-507.

Chapter Six: Medicine on the Assembly-line

1. R. Stevens, *American Medicine and the Public Interest* (New Haven: Yale University Press, 1971), pp98-114.

2. *Ibid.*, p199.

3. P.L. Kendall, "Medical specialization; trends and contributing factors", in R.H. Coombs, C.E. Vincent, *Psychosocial Aspects of Medical Training* (Springfield, Illinois: Charles C. Thomas, 1971), pp449-497.

4. P.L. Kendall, H.C. Selvin, "Tendencies toward specialization in medical training", in R.K. Merton, G.G. Reader and P.L. Kendall (eds.), *The Student Physician* (Cambridge, Mass: Harvard University Press, 1957), pp153-176.

5. R.E. Coker Jr., N. Miller, K.W. Black, T. Donnelly, "The medical stu-

dent, specialization and general practice", *North Carolina Medical Journal* 21 (1960): 96-101.

6. P.L. Kendall, H.C. Selvin, *op.cit.*

7. R. Stevens, *Medical Practice in Modern England* (New Haven: Yale University Press, 1966) pp323-324.

8. P.L. Kendall, *op.cit.*

9. R. Stevens, *Medical Practice in Modern England, op.cit.*, pp183-211.

10. *Ibid.*, pp323-368.

11. A.L. Cochrane, "World health problems", *Canadian Public Health Association Journal* 66, no.4 (1975): 280-287.

12. E. Vayda, "A comparison of surgical rates in Canada and in England and Wales", *New England Journal of Medicine* 289 (1973): 1224-1229.

13. D.L. Sackett et al., "The Burlington randomized trial of the nurse practitioner: health outcomes of patients", *Annals of Internal Medicine* 80, no.2 (1974): 137-142; and A.L. Komaroff et al., "Protocols for physician assistants: management of diabetes and hypertension", *New England Journal of Medicine* 290 (1974): 307-312.

14. D. Rutstein, *The Coming Revolution in Medicine* (Cambridge, Mass.: MIT Press, 1967).

15. Harvard University, "Program on technology and society", *Fourth Annual Report* (Cambridge, Mass: Harvard University Press, 1968).

16. W.A. Knaus, S.A. Schroeder, D.O. Davis, "Impact of new technology: the CT scanner", *Medical Care* 15 (1977): 533-542.

17. H.V. Fineberg, G.S. Parker, L.A. Pearlman, "CT scanners: distribution and planning status in the United States", *New England Journal of Medicine* 297 (1977): 216-218.

18. C.C Korvin, R.H. Pearce, J. Stanley, "Admissions screening: clinical benefits", *Annals of Internal Medicine* 83 (1975): 197-203.

19. A.L. Cochrane, *Effectiveness and efficiency, random reflections on health services* (The Nuffield Provincial Hospitals Trust, 1972), p43.

20. J. Avorn, "The future of doctoring", *The Atlantic Monthly* (November 1974), pp71-79.

21. *Ibid.*, p72.

22. W.V. Slack, C.W. Slack, "Patient-Computer Dialogue", *New England Journal of Medicine* 286 (1972): 1304-1309; and J.S. Maxmen, *The Post-Physician Era: medicine in the 21st century* (New York: John Wiley and Sons), pp48-92.

23. W.B. Dunkman, J.K. Perloff, J.A. Castor, J.C. Shelburne, "Medical perspectives in coronary artery surgery — a caveat", *Annals of Internal Medicine* 81 (1974): 817-837.

24. H.G. Mather, W.G. Pearson, K.L.Q. Read et al., "Acute myocardial infarction, home and hospital treatment", *British Medical Journal* 3 (1971):

334-338; and A.L. Cochrane, *Effectiveness and Efficiency, op.cit.*, pp50-54.

25. E. Krause, "Health and the politics of technology", *Inquiry* 8, no. 3 (September 1971): 51-59.

26. J.D. Hill, J.R. Hampton, J.R.A. Mitchell, "A randomized trial of home-versus-hospital management for patients with suspected myocardial infarction", *Lancet* 1 (1978): 837.

27. "The medical industrial complex", *Health/PAC Bulletin*, November 1969.

28. M.J. Murray, "The pharmaceutical industry: a study in corporate power", *International Journal of Health Services* 4, no.4 (1974): 625-640; and B. Ehrenreich, J. Ehrenreich (eds.), *American Health Empire: Power, Profit, Politics* (New York: Random House, 1970), pp95-123.

29. R. Seidenberg, "Drug advertising and perception of mental illness", *Mental Hygiene* 55, no.1 (January 1971): 21-31.

30. N. Doherty, "Excess profits in the drug industry and their effects on consumer expenditures", *Inquiry* 10 (September 1973): 19-30.

31. S.A. Miller, *White Paper on Health Policy* (Winnipeg: Government of Manitoba, 1973).

32. W.M. Siebert, *Proceedings of the First Conference on Electronics in Medicine* (New York: McGraw-Hill, 1969).

33. A.L. Cochrane, *Effectiveness and Efficiency, op.cit.*

34. H.M. Spiro, "Visceral Viewpoints: My Kingdom for a Camera — some comments on medical technology", *New England Journal of Medicine* 291 (1974): 1070-1072.

35. L. Mumford, *The Myth of the Machine*, vol.2: *The Pentagon of Power* (New York: Columbia University Press, 1970).

36. K. Marx, *The Economic and Philosophic Manuscripts of 1844*, trans. M. Mulligan (New York: International Publishers, 1964), pp147, 149.

37. *Ibid.*, p151.

38. E. Krause, *op.cit.*, p54.

39. K. Marx, *op.cit.*, p139fn.

40. R. John, D. Kimmelman et al., "Public Health Care in Cuba", *Social Policy* (Jan./Feb. 1971), pp41-46; and C. Vukmanovie, "Decentralized socialism: medical care in Yugoslavia", *International Journal of Health Services* 2, no.1 (1972): 35-44.

Chapter Seven: Doctor Talk

1. B.M. Korsch, E.K. Gozzi, V. Francis, "Gaps in doctor-patient communication, 1. Doctor-patient interaction and patient satisfaction", *Pediatrics* 42, no.5 (1970): 855-871.

2. C.M. Boyle, "Difference between patients' and doctors' interpretation

of some common medical terms", *British Medical Journal* 2 (1970): 286-289.

3. B.M. Korsch et al: *op.cit.*

4. *Ibid.*

5. R.E. Reynolds, T.W. Rice, "Attitudes of medical interns towards patients and health professionals", *Journal of Health and Social Behaviour* 12 (1971): 307-311; and E. Mumford, *Interns, From Students to Physicians* (Cambridge, Mass.: Harvard University Press, 1970), pp207-209.

6. C.E. Weise, S.F. Price, "The Benzodinzepines — patterns of use", *Bibliographic Series,* no.9 (Addiction Research Foundation, Toronto, Ont., 1975).

Chapter Eight: Alienation and Authoritarianism in Medicine

1. M. Horkheimer, *The Eclipse of Reason* (New York: Oxford University Press, 1947), p187. ℬ 3Ͻ7ዒ. ዞ8ዓ7ᇀ 3

2. V. Navarro, "The Political Economy of Medical Care: an explanation of the composition, nature and function of the present health sector of the United States", *International Journal of Health Services* 5, no.1 (1975): 65-94.

3. I.D. Illich, *Medical Nemesis: The expropriation of health* (New York: Pantheon, 1975). ᖇᕼ ዛI 8. Ɔዛዛ l98ᘋ science

4. I. Meszaros, *Marx's Theory of Alienation* (London: The Merlin Press, 1970); and R. Schacht, *Alienation* (New York: Doubleday and Company, 1970).

5. B. Ollman, *Alienation: Marx's Concept of Man in Capitalist Society* (Cambridge: Cambridge University Press, 1971), p131.

6. K. Marx, Preface to *A Contribution to the Critique of Political Economy,* trans. M. Mulligan (New York: International Publishers, 1970), p20.

7. I. Meszaros, *op.cit.,* pp173-174.

8. *Ibid.*

9. Harry Braverman, *Labour and Monopoly Capital: The Degradation of Work in the Twentieth Century* (New York: Monthly Review Press, 1974).

10. I. Meszaros, *op.cit.*

11. *Ibid.*

12. K. Marx, *The Economic and Philosophic Manuscripts of 1844,* trans. M. Mulligan (New York: International Publishers, 1964), pp110-111.

13. G. Lukacs, *History and Class Consciousness,* trans. R. Livingstone (London: The Merlin Press, 1971), p89.

14. *Ibid.,* pp86-90.

15. *Ibid.,* p89.

16. *Ibid.*, p50.
17. *Ibid.*, p76.
18. K. Marx, *The Economic and Philosophic Manuscripts of 1844, op.cit.*, p108.
19. K. Marx *A Contribution to the Critique of Political Economy, op.cit.*, pp195-199.
20. K. Marx, *The Economic and Philosophic Manuscripts of 1844, op.cit.*, p147.
21. *Ibid.*, p116.
22. *Ibid.*, p114.
23. G. Lukacs, *op.cit.*, pp14-15.
24. "The miners: a special case", (editorial) *The Lancet* 1 (1974): 81-82.
25. H.B. Waitzkin, B. Waterman, *The Exploitation of Illness in Capitalist Society* (New York: Bobbs Merrill, 1974), p68. RA 418. W34
26. *Ibid.*, p75.
27. E. Fromm, *Escape from Freedom* (New York: Holt, Rinehart and Winston, 1941), pp154-157.
28. *Ibid.*, p168.
29. E. Fromm, *The Sane Society* (Greenwich, Conn: Fawcett, 1955), p90.
30. E. Fromm, *Escape from Freedom, op.cit.*, p108.
31. *Ibid.*, pp101-102.
32. *Ibid.*, pp255-257.
33. *Ibid.*, p155.
34. T.W. Adorno et al., *The Authoritarian Personality* (New York: Harper and Brothers, 1950), pp759-760.
35. E. Fromm, *The Anatomy of Human Destructiveness* (New York: Holt, Rinehart and Winston, 1973), pp297-298.
36. *Ibid.*
37. R. Christie, R.K. Merton, "Procedures for the sociological study of the value climate in medical schools", *Journal of Medical Education* 33 (1958): 247-256.
38. E. Fromm, *The Anatomy of Human Destructiveness, op.cit.*, p290.